Diabetic Desserts for Beginners

Easy Low Sugar Recipes for Losing Weight and Healthy Living, Great for Beginners

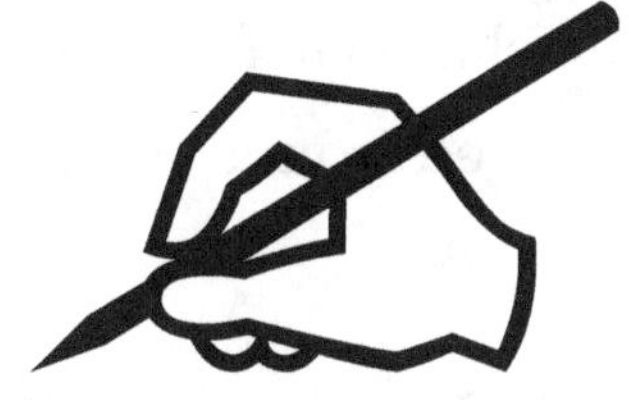

By

Felicity Bath

CONTENTS

Introduction

Congratulations on purchasing your copy of *Diabetic Desserts for Beginners,* and thank you for doing so. This cookbook will guide you to ways of enjoying diabetic desserts for beginners or pros, and it will help you prepare sugar-free or low-sugar desserts with simple and easy-to-find ingredients.

If you have prediabetes or diabetes, your physician will probably suggest you meet with a professional to create a balanced meal plan. You need to keep your blood sugar at an acceptable level. Doing so helps prevent high blood pressure, helps eliminate heart disease risk, and keeps your weight in line with your frame and activity levels.

As you consume extra fat and calories, your body will respond with a rise in your blood glucose. Always follow a diabetes diet, which is based on eating three, regularly scheduled meals daily.

Suggested Foods

Dietary fiber moderates how your body digests the food you eat and helps control blood sugar levels. Choose healthy carbohydrates and foods containing fiber, including:

- ❖ Low-fat dairy products (cheese & milk)
- ❖ Legumes (peas & beans)
- ❖ Whole grains
- ❖ Fruits
- ❖ Vegetables
- ❖ Nuts
- ❖ Whole grains

Two times each week, prepare a delicious platter of fish to provide essential omega-3 fatty acids. *Avoid* the king mackerel since it has high levels of mercury. Incorporate a serving of sardines for a snack or a piece of salmon for dinner.

Foods containing polyunsaturated and monounsaturated fats *can* help lower cholesterol levels. Enjoy a few nuts, olives, and avocados. Using oils derived from olives, nuts, peanuts, or canola are good options.

Foods to Avoid

Consider these categories:

- ❖ *Cholesterol* is definitely an enemy on the top spot from elements included in animal proteins and high-fat dairy (organ meats, such as liver or egg yolks). Set your goals by not exceeding more than 200 milligrams (mg) daily.
- ❖ *Trans fats* include processed baked goods, snacks, stick margarine, and shortening.
- ❖ *Saturated fats* include high-fat dairy and animal products, proteins (sausage, bacon, hot dogs, beef & butter). Consume less palm kernel and coconut oils.
- ❖ *Sodium*. Consume under 2,300 mg daily. Add the elements of high blood pressure, and you will further need to lower your intakes.

Each of the recipes has a breakdown of its nutritional values.

Chapter 1

Yogurt Parfait Specialties

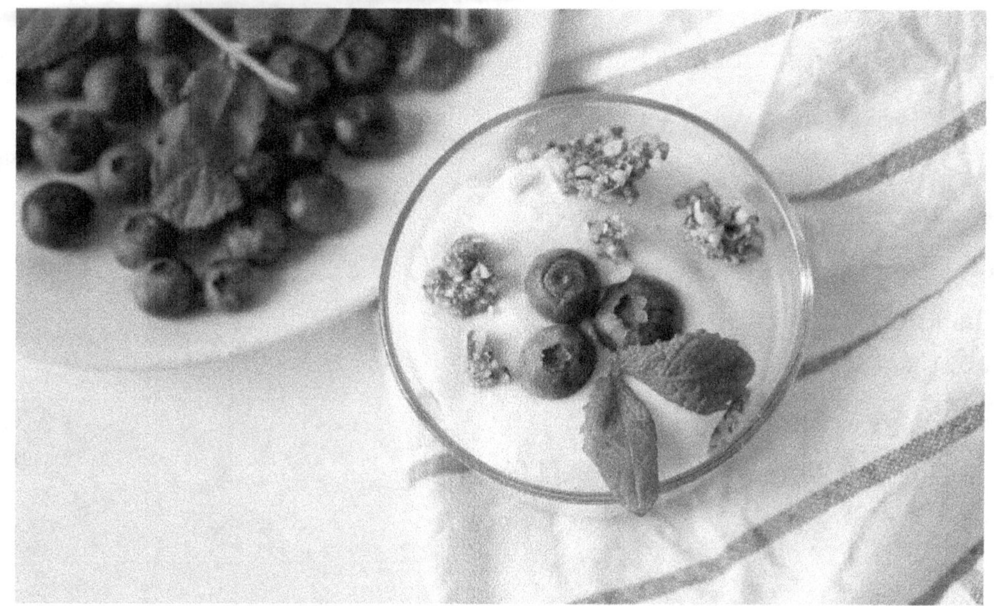

Note; most of the recipes are coded with their diabetic exchanges (DE) when available!

Servings Provided: 4

Time Required: 20 minutes

Macro Counts - Each Serving:

- ❖ Calories: 129
- ❖ Carbs: 27 g
- ❖ Sugar: 17.5 g
- ❖ Fiber: 3.7 g
- ❖ Chol: -0- mg

- ❖ Prot.: 6.4 g
- ❖ Sodium: 75.3 mg
- ❖ Fat Content: 0.4 g (Saturated: -0- g)
  D.E.:
- ❖ Starch: 1
- ❖ Fat: ½
- ❖ Milk: ½

Ingredients Needed:

- ❖ Greek yogurt - fat-free - plain (1 cup)
- ❖ Vanilla (1 tsp.)
- ❖ Honey (2 tbsp.)
- ❖ Fresh raspberries (.5 cup)
- ❖ Lemon peel (.5 tsp.)
- ❖ Fresh blackberries (.5 cup)
- ❖ Fresh blueberries (.5 cup)
- ❖ Multigrain oats & honey cereal (1 cup)
- ❖ Optional Garnish: Lemon peel strips (4 pinches)

Preparation Technique:

1. Finely shred the lemon peel and slice the blackberries.
2. Combine the yogurt with the honey, vanilla, and shredded lemon peel (½ tsp.).
3. Scoop half of the yogurt mixture into four parfait dishes.
4. Garnish the parfait with ½ of the cereal and berries. Repeat the layers.
5. Serve it promptly or cover and chill up to ½ hour. Garnish with lemon peel strips.

Chocolate Pudding Sandwiches

Servings Provided: 3.5 dozen

Time Required: 20 minutes + freeze time

Macro Counts - Each Serving:

- ❖ Calories: 75
- ❖ Sodium: 107 mg
- ❖ Carbs: 12 g
- ❖ Sugar: 6 g
- ❖ Fiber: 1 g
- ❖ Prot.: 1 g
- ❖ Chol: -0- mg
- ❖ Fat Content: 2 g (Saturated: 1 g)
  D.E:
- ❖ Starch: 1
- ❖ Fat: ½

Ingredients Needed:

- ❖ Cold milk - fat-free (1.5 cups)
- ❖ Instant chocolate - Sugar-free pudding mix (1.4 oz. pkg.)
- ❖ Frozen & thawed reduced-fat whipped topping (8 oz. carton)
- ❖ Miniature marshmallows (1 cup)
- ❖ Chocolate wafers (9 oz. pkg. - 2 each)

Preparation Technique:

1. Make the filling by whisking the milk and pudding mix for two minutes. Wait for two minutes and mix in the whipped topping, and lastly, the marshmallows.
2. Spread about two tablespoons of the prepared filling onto the bottom of a wafer (for each sandwich). Add another wafer. Stack the sandwiches in covered containers.
3. Freeze until firm (3 hrs.).
4. Remove the container from the freezer. Thaw it and wait for five minutes before serving.

Mixed Berry Sundaes

Servings Provided: 2

Time Required: 10 minutes

Macro Counts - Each Serving:

- ❖ Calories: 160
- ❖ Carbs: 22 g
- ❖ Fiber: 3 g
- ❖ Sugar: 18 g
- ❖ Chol: -0- mg
- ❖ Fat Content: 5 g (Sat.: -0- g)
- ❖ Protein: 10 g
- ❖ Sodium: 33 mg
  D.E:
- ❖ Starch: 1
- ❖ Fat: 1
- ❖ Fruit: ½

Ingredients Needed:

- ❖ Halved fresh strawberries (.25 cup)
- ❖ Fresh raspberries, blueberries & blackberries (.25 cup each)
- ❖ Honey - divided (3 tsp.)
- ❖ F.F. Greek yogurt - plain (.5 cup)
- ❖ Pomegranate juice (2 tbsp.)
- ❖ Chopped walnuts - toasted (2 tbsp.)

Preparation Technique:

1. Toss the berries and one teaspoon of honey. Spoon the berries into two dessert dishes.
2. Combine the pomegranate juice with the yogurt and remaining honey. Scoop it over the berries. Sprinkle with walnuts and serve.

Vanilla Custard & Berries

Servings Provided: 4

Time Required: 20 minutes + chill time

Macro Counts - Each Serving:

- ❖ With ¼ cup of sauce:
- ❖ Calories: 166
- ❖ Carbs: 16 g
- ❖ Sugar: 11 g
- ❖ Fiber: 4 g
- ❖ Chol: 132 mg
- ❖ Fat Content: 9 g (Saturated: 5 g)
- ❖ Protein: 4 g
- ❖ Sodium: 34 mg
  - **D.E**:
- ❖ Starch: ½
- ❖ Fat: 1 ½
- ❖ Fruit: ½

Ingredients Needed:

- ❖ Half-&-Half cream (1 cup)
- ❖ Egg yolks (2 large)
- ❖ Sugar (2 tbsp.)
- ❖ Vanilla extract (2 tsp.)
- ❖ Fresh berries (2 cups)

Preparation Technique:

1. Use a small heavy saucepan to mix the cream with the egg yolks and sugar. Simmer using the low-temperature setting until the mixture is 'just' thickened and reads at least 160° F/71° C on a thermometer. *Don't boil.*
2. Put the mixture into a mixing container and mix in the vanilla. Pop it into the fridge, covered until it's cold. Serve over fresh berries.

Chapter 2

Smoothies & Frozen Treats

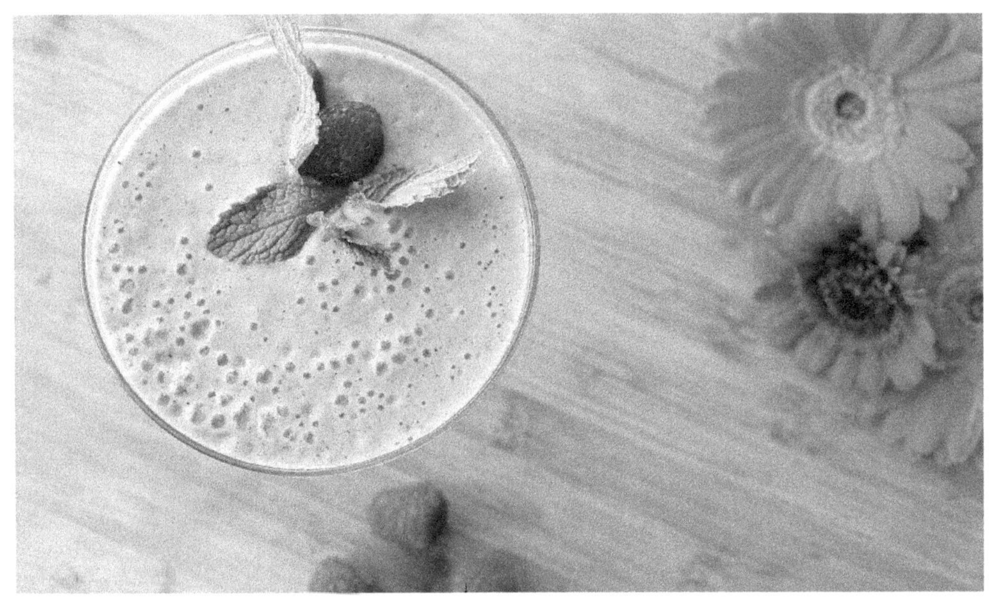

Enjoy a delicious smoothie for breakfast or dessert!

Smoothies

Avocado Chocolate Smoothie - Gluten-Free Vegan

Servings Provided: 2

Time Required: 5 minutes

Macro Counts - Each Serving:

- ❖ Calories: 319
- ❖ Carbs: 12.1 g
- ❖ Fiber: 5.5g
- ❖ Sugar: 2.4 g

- ❖ Chol: -0- mg
- ❖ Protein: 2.3 g
- ❖ Sodium: 180.2 mg
- ❖ Fat Content: 30.6 g (Saturated: 23.4 g)
- ❖ Net Carbs: 6.6 g

Ingredients Needed:

- ❖ Ripe avocado (half of 1)
- ❖ Cocoa powder (3 tbsp.)
- ❖ Coconut milk - full-fat (1 cup)
- ❖ Water (.5 cup/1.2 dl)
- ❖ Lime juice (1 tsp.)
- ❖ Mineral salt (1 pinch)
- ❖ Liquid Stevia (6-7 drops)
- ❖ To Garnish: Fresh mint (as desired)

Preparation Technique:

1. Add all of the ingredients into the blender.
2. Mix using the high-speed setting until it's mixed and creamy. If desired, add more liquid stevia to taste.
3. Top it off using a sprig of fresh mint and serve.

Berry Smoothie in a Bowl

Servings Provided: 2

Time Required: 5 minutes

Macro Counts - Each Serving:

- ❖ Calories: 166
- ❖ Carbs: 4.1 g
- ❖ Sugar: 1.2 g
- ❖ Fiber: 3.3 g
- ❖ Chol: -0- mg
- ❖ Prot.: 17.6 g
- ❖ Sodium: 49.1 mg
- ❖ Fat Content: 9.2 g (Saturated: 6 g)
- ❖ Net Carbs: 0.8 g

Ingredients Needed:

- ❖ Unsweetened almond milk (.5 cup/125 ml)
- ❖ Chopped strawberries (2 oz./50 g)
- ❖ Crushed ice (3 cups/750 ml)
- ❖ Pea/vanilla protein powder (.33 cup/40 g)
- ❖ Psyllium husk powder (.5 tsp.)
- ❖ Coconut oil (1 tbsp.)
- ❖ Liquid Stevia (5 – 10 drops)

Preparation Technique:

1. Put the ice cubes in a blender and allow them to sit for five minutes. You want them to melt slightly, so the blender has some traction.
2. Add the rest of the fixings and mix until it's light pink and creamy.
3. Pour it into a serving bowl and top it off using desired toppings.

Delicious Snickers Smoothie

Servings Provided: 1

Time Required: 5 minutes

Macro Counts - Each Serving:

- ❖ Calories: 309
- ❖ Carbs: 35.2 g
- ❖ Fiber: 14.8 g
- ❖ Protein: 18.4 g
- ❖ Fat Content: 11.2 g

Ingredients Needed:

- ❖ Almond milk - unsweetened (1 cup)
- ❖ Unsweetened - plain yogurt/plain kefir (.5 cup)
- ❖ Stevia - ex. Sweet Leaf brand (2 packets)
- ❖ Unsweetened cocoa powder (1 tbsp.)
- ❖ English Toffee stevia (5 drops)
- ❖ Creamy peanut/almond butter & no sugar added (1 heaping tbsp.)
- ❖ PaleoFiber powder/chia seed/ground flaxseed meal (1 tbsp.)
- ❖ Collagen hydrolysate/Vanilla protein powder of your choice (1 tbsp.)
- ❖ Vanilla extract (.5 tsp.)

Preparation Technique:

1. Toss the fixings into your blender.
2. Set using the high setting, pulsing until thoroughly combined.

The Greenie

Servings Provided: 3 medium

Time Required: 12 minutes

Macro Counts - Each Serving:

- ❖ Calories: 123
- ❖ Carbs: 31 g
- ❖ Sugar: 17 g
- ❖ Fiber: 5 g
- ❖ Prot.: 2 g
- ❖ Sodium: 30 mg

Ingredients Needed:

- ❖ Water (1.5 cups/375g)
- ❖ Fresh kale or spinach (2 cups/134g)
- ❖ Fresh mint (.5 cup/22.5g)
- ❖ Ripe green pear (1)
- ❖ Chilled green or Moscato grapes (20)
- ❖ Ripe green apple (1)
- ❖ Ice cubes (12)
- ❖ Cinnamon (.75 tsp)
- ❖ Stevia (1 tsp.) or Agave nectar (1 tbsp./ as desired)
- ❖ Lime (1 - juiced, or more to taste)
- ❖ Note: Use organic produce if available

Preparation Technique:

1. Remove the core from the apples and pear and chop them into chunks. Roughly chop the kale/spinach and mint.
2. Pour the cold water into the blender with a small handful of the apple and pear chunks. Blend till the mixture is thoroughly liquified. Continue adding them until they are gone.
3. Add the greens and mint the same way. Blend in batches if needed until all of the greens have been incorporated. Add the grapes, ice cubes, agave/stevia, cinnamon, and lime juice.

4. Blend the mixture until the ice cubes are thoroughly crushed, and the mixture is smooth (1 min.).
5. Serve for an energized day!
6. Note: Please be sure to follow the steps in the order suggested. Otherwise, they won't blend properly.

Strawberry Smoothie - Vegetarian

Servings Provided: 1

Time Required: 5 minutes

Macro Counts - Each Serving:

- ❖ Calories: 167
- ❖ Carbs: 11 g
- ❖ Sugar: 6 g
- ❖ Fiber: 2 g
- ❖ Chol: 8 mg
- ❖ Prot.: 16 g
- ❖ Sodium: 161 mg
- ❖ Fat Content: 6 g (Saturated: 1 g)

Ingredients Needed:

- ❖ Strawberries (5 medium)
- ❖ Unsweetened almond/soy milk (1 cup)
- ❖ Greek-style yogurt - L.F. (.5 cup)
- ❖ Ice (6 cubes)

Preparation Technique:

1. Toss each of the ingredients into a blender, mixing until creamy.
2. Serve in a chilled glass with a fresh strawberry!

Strawberry Banana Smoothie

Servings Provided: 1

Time Required: 5 minutes

Macro Counts - Each Serving:

- ❖ Calories: 276
- ❖ Fiber: 14.3 g
- ❖ Carbs: 44.7 g
- ❖ Prot.: 16.7 g
- ❖ Sodium: mg
- ❖ Fat Content: 2.6 g

Ingredients Needed:

- ❖ Almond milk - unsweetened (1 cup)
- ❖ Unsweetened plain yogurt/unsweetened plain kefir (.5 cup)
- ❖ Stevia (2 packets)
- ❖ Banana (¼ of 1 small)
- ❖ Fresh or frozen strawberries (.5 cup)
- ❖ Paleo Fiber powder/ground flaxseed meal/chia seed (1 tbsp.)
- ❖ Collagen hydrolysate/vanilla protein powder of your choice (1 tbsp.)
- ❖ Vanilla extract (.5 tsp.)

Preparation Technique:

1. Toss all of the fixings into a blender.
2. Mix using the high-speed setting.

Strawberry Pineapple Smoothie

Servings Provided: 1

Time Required: 5 minutes

Macro Counts - Each Serving:

- ❖ Calories: 255
- ❖ Carbs: 39 g
- ❖ Sugar: 24 g
- ❖ Fiber: 7.8 g
- ❖ Protein: 5.6 g
- ❖ Sodium: 168.4 mg
- ❖ Fat Content: 11.1 g (Saturated: 1.1 g)
  D.E.:
- ❖ Fat: 2
- ❖ Fruit: 2 ½

Ingredients Needed:

- ❖ Frozen strawberries (1 cup)
- ❖ Freshly chopped pineapple (1 cup)
- ❖ Chilled unsweetened almond milk (.75 cup + more if needed)
- ❖ Almond butter (1 tbsp.)

Preparation Technique:

1. Toss the pineapple, strawberries, almond butter, and almond milk into a blender.
2. Pulse until it's creamy smooth, adding more almond milk, if needed, for desired consistency.
3. Serve promptly.

Other Unique Frozen Treats

When you prepare ice pops, you can use molds such as the ones provided by Tupperware or use a paper cup. Cover the cup with a piece of aluminum foil. Poke a wooden stick/handle in through the foil and freeze the pop.

Some of the recipes will suggest using an ice cream maker. In its place, use a shallow metal pan or ice cube trays to freeze the pops. Pop it in the freezer until firm (6 hrs.). Once it is frozen, use a mallet to break it apart. Pop it into the food processor to mix until creamy smooth.

Berry White Ice Pops

Servings Provided: 10

Time Required: 10 minutes + freeze time

Macro Counts - Each Serving:

- ❖ Calories: 51
- ❖ Carbs: 8 g
- ❖ Sugar: 6 g
- ❖ Fiber: 2 g
- ❖ Chol: 4 mg
- ❖ Prot.: 2 g
- ❖ Sodium: 19 mg
- ❖ Fat Content: 2 g (Saturated: 1 g)
  D.E.:
- ❖ Starch: ½

Ingredients Needed:

- ❖ Whole milk - divided (1.75 cups)
- ❖ Honey (1-2 tbsp.)
- ❖ Vanilla extract (.25 tsp.)
- ❖ Blueberries - fresh (1 cup)
- ❖ Raspberries - fresh (1.5 cups)
- ❖ Paper cups or freezer pop molds & sticks (10 @ about 6 tbsp. each)

Preparation Technique:

1. Pour the water into a safe container and warm ¼ cup of milk in the microwave. Stir in the honey and rest of the milk (1.5 cups), and vanilla.
2. Portion the berries into the molds, and pour milk into the mixture. Place the tops onto the molds with holders.
3. Pop them in the freezer until they are solid to serve.

Chocolate Greek Yogurt Ice Cream

Servings Provided: 1

Time Required: 2 hours

Macro Counts - Each Serving:

- ❖ Calories: 127
- ❖ Carbs: 8.1 g
- ❖ Sugar: 4.4 g
- ❖ Chol: 9.7 mg
- ❖ Protein: 20.1 g
- ❖ Sodium: 150 mg
- ❖ Fat Content: 2.2 g (Saturated: 0.4 g)
- ❖ Net Carbs: 5.6 g

Ingredients Needed:

- ❖ Almond milk - unsweetened (.5 cup or 120 ml)
- ❖ Fat-free Greek yogurt (2.5 oz./75 g)
- ❖ Vanilla protein powder (.5 oz./15 g)
- ❖ Unsweetened cocoa powder (1 tsp.)
- ❖ Stevia (2 tbsp./to taste)
- ❖ Vanilla extract (1 tsp.)
- ❖ Optional: Almonds & berries
- ❖ Useful: Blender/whisk

Preparation Technique:

1. Blend the yogurt with the protein powder, stevia, cocoa, and almond milk. Place the mixture in your freezer or ice cream machine.
2. If making in the freezer, remove the ice cream out after an hour and gently stir using a spoon to avoid a large ice block. Repeat every ½ hour until the ice cream has the right consistency (2 hours total).
3. After the waiting time has elapsed, take the ice cream from the freezer five to ten minutes before you are prepared to serve it.

Chunky Banana Cream Freeze

Servings Provided: 3 cups

Time Required: 15 minutes + freeze time

Macro Counts - Each Serving:

- ½ cup per portion:
- Calories: 181
- Carbs: 29 g
- Sugar: 16 g
- Fiber: 4 g
- Chol: -0- mg
- Prot.: 3 g
- Fat Content: 7 g (Saturated: 2 g)
- Sodium: 35 mg
  D.E:
- Starch: ½
- Fat: 1
- Fruit: 1

Ingredients Needed:

- Bananas - peeled & frozen (5 medium)
- Unsweetened coconut - finely shredded (2 tbsp.)
- Almond milk (.33 cup)
- Vanilla extract (1 tsp.)
- Creamy peanut butter (2 tbsp.)
- Chopped walnuts (.25 cup)
- Raisins (3 tbsp.)

Preparation Technique:

1. Place the bananas, peanut butter, milk, vanilla, and coconut in a food processor. Close the lid and blend the mixture.

2. Pour it into a freezer container, and fold in the walnuts and raisins. Freeze for two to four hours before serving.

Frozen Berry & Yogurt Swirls

Servings Provided: 10 pops

Time Required: 15 minutes + freeze time

Macro Counts - Each Serving:

- ❖ Calories: 60
- ❖ Carbs: 9 g
- ❖ Sugar: 8 g
- ❖ Fiber: 1 g
- ❖ Chol: -0- mg
- ❖ Prot.: 6 g
- ❖ Fat Content: -0-g
- ❖ Sodium: 28 mg
- ❖ **D.E**:
- ❖ Starch: 1

Ingredients Needed:

- ❖ Plastic or paper cups (10 @ 3 oz. each)
- ❖ Honey Greek yogurt - fat-free (2.75 cups)
- ❖ Fresh berries - mixed (1 cup)
- ❖ Water (.25 cup)
- ❖ Sugar (2 tbsp.)
- ❖ Wooden pop sticks (10)

Preparation Technique:

1. Fill each cup with yogurt (¼ cup).
2. Prepare the food processor. Toss in the berries, water, and sugar. Swirl it until the berries are thoroughly chopped.
3. Scoop 1.5 tablespoons of the berry mixture into each cup. Gently stir using a popsicle stick to swirl.

Top each of the cups with foil and add the pop sticks in through foil. Freeze until firm.

Grab any time for a delicious treat!

Frozen Yogurt Fruit Pops

Servings Provided: 1 dozen

Time Required: 15 minutes + freeze time

Macro Counts - Each Serving:

- Calories: 60
- Carbs: 13 g
- Sugar: 10 g
- Fiber: 1 g
- Chol: 2 mg
- Prot.: 2 g
- Sodium: 23 mg
- Fat Content: 1 g (Saturated: -0- g)
  D.E:
- Starch: 1

Ingredients Needed:

- Raspberry yogurt (2.25 cups)
- Lemon juice (2 tbsp.)
- Ripe bananas (2 medium)
- Freezer pop mold/paper cups (12 @ 3 oz. each) and wooden pop sticks

Preparation Technique:

1. Cut the banana into chunks.
2. Scoop the yogurt, lemon juice, and bananas into a blender. Put the top on the blender and mix until it's creamy.
3. Scoop the prepared mixture into the cups and add the holders. Freeze until they are firm.

Hazelnut Chocolate Soy Pops

Servings Provided: 8

Time Required: 10 minutes + freeze time

Macro Counts - Each Serving:

- ❖ Calories: 94
- ❖ Carbs: 11 g
- ❖ Sugar: 10 g
- ❖ Sodium: 33 mg
- ❖ Fiber: -0- g
- ❖ Chol: -0- mg
- ❖ Fat Content: 4 g (Saturated: 1 g)
- ❖ Protein: 4 g
  D.E:
- ❖ Starch: 1
- ❖ Fat: ½

Ingredients Needed:

- ❖ Soy milk - vanilla (1 cup)
- ❖ Fat-free milk (.5 cup)
- ❖ Vanilla Greek yogurt - fat-free (.75 cup)
- ❖ Nutella (1/3 cup)
- ❖ Paper cups/pop molds (8 @ 3 ounces each) & wooden pop sticks

Preparation Technique:

1. Pour the milk, yogurt, and Nutella into a blender.
2. Securely close the top and mix until it's creamy. Scoop it into the holders and seal the tops with foil, adding the sticks.
3. Freeze until firm.

Lemon-Apricot Fruit Pops

Servings Provided: 6

Time Required: 15 minutes + freeze time

Macro Counts - Each Serving:

- ❖ Calories: 31
- ❖ Carbs: 8 g
- ❖ Fiber: 1 g
- ❖ Sugar: 6 g
- ❖ Chol: -0- mg
- ❖ Sodium: -0- mg
- ❖ Fat Content: -0- g (Saturated: -0- g)
- ❖ Prot.: -0- g
  D.E:
- ❖ Fruit: ½

Ingredients Needed:

- ❖ Orange juice (.25 cup)
- ❖ Grated lemon zest (1 tsp.)
- ❖ Sugar (4 tsp.)
- ❖ Lemon juice (.25 cup)
- ❖ Fresh apricots (1 cup/4-5 medium)
- ❖ Ice cubes (.5 cup)
  ****
- ❖ Optional: 1 teaspoon minced fresh mint (1 tsp.)
- ❖ Molds & sticks for the pops (6 @ 6 tbsp. each)

Preparation Technique:

1. Slice the apricots and make the juice and zest from the lemon.
2. Toss the first six fixings into a blender (up to the line**); cover and process until blended. Add in freshly minced mint.
3. Pour the mixture into molds and freeze until firm.

Patriotic Pops

Servings Provided: 12

Time Required: 15 minutes + freeze time

Macro Counts - Each Serving:

- Calories: 55
- Carbs: 11 g
- Sugar: 10 g
- Chol: 2 mg
- Fiber: 1 g
- Prot.: 2 g
- Fat Content: 1 g (Saturated: -0- g)
- Sodium: 24 mg
  D.E:
- Starch: 1

Ingredients Needed:

- Vanilla yogurt - divided (1.75 cups)
- Honey - divided (2 tbsp.)
- Fresh strawberries - sliced & divided (1.25 cups)
- Frozen or fresh blueberries - thawed & divided (1.25 cups)
- Freezer popsicle molds/paper cups (12 @ 3 oz. each) & wooden pop sticks

Preparation Technique:

1. Measure and add one tablespoon honey, two tablespoons yogurt, and one cup strawberries in a blender. Place the lid on tightly and process until blended. Pour it into a small, holding container.
2. Chop the rest of the strawberries and add them to the mixture.
3. Use a blender to process the rest of the honey with two tablespoons of yogurt and one cup of blueberries. Transfer them to another container. Fold in the rest of the blueberries.
4. Prepare the molds. Scoop the strawberry mixture (1 tbsp.), yogurt (2 tbsp.), and blueberry mixture (1 tbsp.).
5. Top with the popsicle sticks or cover the cups with a layer of foil. Freeze until firm.

Peach Sorbet

Servings Provided: 8

Time Required: 4 hours 45 minutes

Macro Counts - Each Serving:

- ❖ Calories: 94
- ❖ Carbs: 24g
- ❖ Fiber: 1.1 g
- ❖ Sugar: 22.6 g
- ❖ Chol: -0- mg
- ❖ Prot.: 0.7 g
- ❖ Sodium: 3.3 mg
- ❖ Fat Content: 0.2 g (Saturated: -0- g)
  D.E.:
- ❖ Fruit: ½
- ❖ Other Carbohydrate: 1 ½

Ingredients Needed:

- ❖ White grape juice (1 cup)
- ❖ Frozen/fresh ripe peaches (about 4/4 cups)
- ❖ Lemon juice (1 tbsp.)
- ❖ Sugar (.5 cup)
- ❖ Also Needed: Ice cream maker**

Preparation Technique:

1. Set up the food processor. Quarter and puree the peaches.
2. Whisk both of the juices and sugar in a saucepan. Warm it using the medium-temperature setting, stirring until it's liquified.
3. Combine and chill the fixings (syrup and fruit puree) in the fridge (4 hs.).
4. Add the sorbet mixture into an ice cream maker.
5. It will be delicious for up to one week. Be sure to slightly soften it before serving.

Raspberry-Banana Soft-Serve

Servings Provided: 2.5 cups/.5 cup portions

Time Required: 10 minutes + freeze time

Macro Counts - Each Serving:

- ❖ Calories: 104
- ❖ Carbs: 26 g
- ❖ Sugar: 15 g
- ❖ Fiber: 2 g
- ❖ Chol: 1 mg
- ❖ Prot.: 2 g
- ❖ Sodium: 15 mg
- ❖ Fat Content: 0 g (Saturated: 0 g)
  D.E:
- ❖ Fruit: 1
- ❖ Starch: ½

Ingredients Needed:

- ❖ Ripe bananas (4 medium)
- ❖ Fat-free plain yogurt (.5 cup)
- ❖ Maple syrup (1-2 tbsp.)
- ❖ Frozen unsweetened raspberries (.5 cup)
- ❖ Optional: Fresh raspberries

Preparation Technique:

1. Thinly slice the bananas and transfer them into a large plastic zipper-type freezer bag. Arrange the slices in a single layer; freeze overnight.
2. Finely chop the bananas in a food processor.
3. Mix in the yogurt, maple syrup, and raspberries. Pulse the mixture a few times just until smooth, scraping sides as needed.
4. Serve immediately, adding fresh berries as desired.

Strawberry Lemonade Popsicles

Servings Provided: 6

Time Required: 5 minutes + chill time of 3 hours

Macro Counts - Each Serving:

- ❖ Calories: 73
- ❖ Carbs: 14.2 g
- ❖ Sugar: 8 g
- ❖ Fiber: 2 g
- ❖ Chol: 1.7 mg
- ❖ Protein: 3.5 g
- ❖ Sodium: 67 mg
- ❖ Fat Content: 0.5 g (Saturated: 0.1 g)
- ❖ Net Carbs: 12.2 g

Ingredients Needed:

- ❖ Old-fashioned oats (.25 cup/22 g)
- ❖ Low fat cottage cheese (4 oz./115 g)
- ❖ Strawberries (1.5 lb./680 g)
- ❖ Lemon juice (4 oz./about 4 lemons/115 g)
- ❖ Liquid Stevia (5 drops)
- ❖ Essential: Food processor or high-powered blender

Preparation Technique:

1. Pulse the oats until they're powdery.
2. Add the cottage cheese, strawberries, stevia, and lemon juice.
3. Pulse the mixture until smooth. Don't add any liquid!
4. Prepare the six molds and freeze until firm (3 hrs.).

Strawberry-Rhubarb Ice Pops

Servings Provided: 8

Time Required: 25 minutes + cool time

Macro Counts - Each Serving:

- ❖ Calories: 72
- ❖ Carbs: 16 g
- ❖ Fiber: 1 g
- ❖ Sugar: 14 g
- ❖ Sodium: 18 mg
- ❖ Prot.: 2 g
- ❖ Chol: 2 mg
- ❖ Fat Content: -0- g (Saturated: -0- g)
  D.E:
- ❖ Starch: 1

Ingredients Needed:

- ❖ Chopped fresh or frozen rhubarb (3 cups)
- ❖ Sugar (.25 cup)
- ❖ Water (3 tbsp.)
- ❖ Strawberry yogurt (1 cup)
- ❖ Unsweetened applesauce (.5 cup)
- ❖ Finely chopped fresh strawberries (.25 cup)
- ❖ Optional: Red food coloring(2 drops)
- ❖ Paper cups/freezer pop molds (8 @ 3 ounces each) and wooden sticks

Preparation Technique:

1. Slice the rhubarb into ½-inch cuts and mix with the water and sugar in a big saucepan. Once boiling, reduce the temperature setting to simmer, uncovered, until thick and blended (10-15 min.). Remove 3/4 cup mixture to a bowl; cool completely. (Save remaining rhubarb for another use.)

2. Add the yogurt, applesauce, and strawberries to the bowl; stir until blended. If desired, tint with food coloring.
3. Fill each mold or cup with about 1/4 cup of the rhubarb mixture.
4. Top the molds with holders and top cups with a layer of foil. Push the sticks through the foil. Freeze until they are firm.

Strawberry Sorbet Sensation

Servings Provided: 8

Time Required: 20 minutes + freeze time

Macro Counts - Each Serving:

- Calories: 153
- Carbs: 27 g
- Sugar: 18 g
- Fiber: 2 g
- Chol: 1 mg
- Prot.: 1 g
- Fat Content: 3 g (Saturated: 3 g)
- Sodium: 163 mg
  D.E:
- Starch: 2
- Fat: ½

Ingredients Needed:

- Strawberry sorbet (2 cups)
- Cold milk- fat-free (1 cup)
- Instant vanilla pudding mix - sugar-free (1 oz. pkg.)
- Reduced-fat whipped topping (frozen 8 oz. carton)
- Sliced fresh strawberries
- Also Suggested: 8x4-inch loaf pan

Preparation Technique:

1. Thaw the whipped topping.
2. Line the loaf pan with plastic wrap. Slightly soften the sorbet and add it to the pan. Freeze it for about 15 minutes.
3. Meanwhile, whisk the pudding mix with the milk for two minutes. It will be soft-set soon (2 min.). Mix and add the thawed topping over the sorbet. Cover the container to freeze and set for four hours to overnight.

4. Transfer the pan to the countertop to slightly thaw before serving (10-15 min.). Flip and invert the dessert onto a plate. Discard the plastic and slice the sorbet. Lastly, slice the strawberries and sprinkle them over the top to serve.

Chapter 3

Muffins

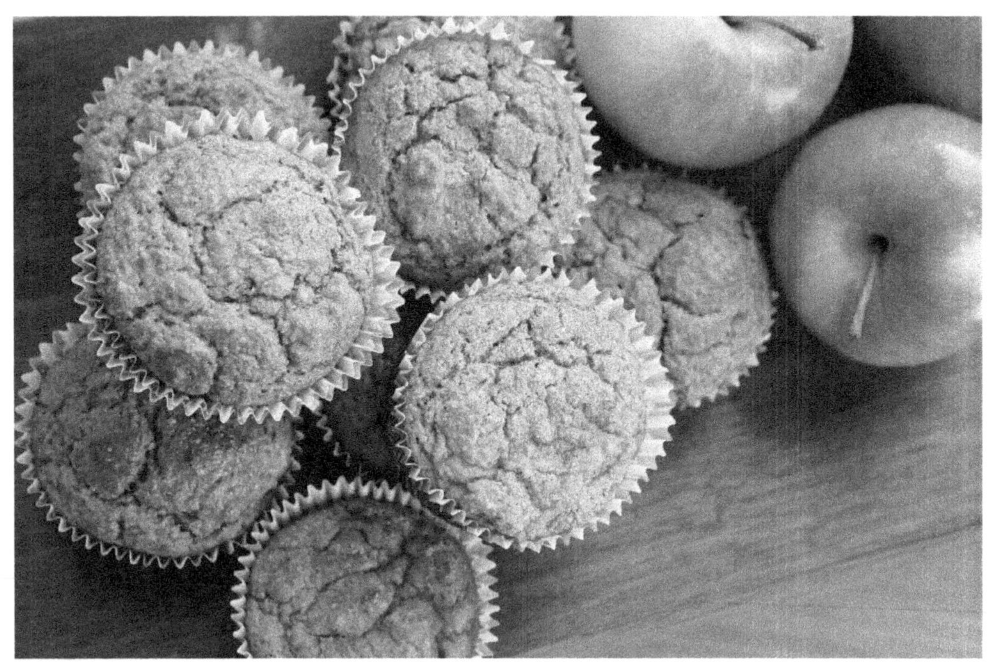

Servings Provided: 6

Time Required: 30-35 minutes

Macro Counts - Each Serving:

- ❖ Calories: 270
- ❖ Carbs: 34 g
- ❖ Sugar: 17 g
- ❖ Fiber: 3 g
- ❖ Chol: 30 mg
- ❖ Prot.: 5 g

- ❖ Sodium: 360 mg
- ❖ Fat Content: 14 g (Saturated: 1.4 g)

Ingredients Needed:

- ❖ Bak. powder (1 tsp.)
- ❖ Flour - whole wheat (1 cup)
- ❖ Cinnamon - ground (1 tsp.)
- ❖ Bak. soda (.25 tsp.)
- ❖ Kosher salt (.5 tsp.)
  ****
- ❖ Canola oil (.25 cup)
- ❖ Brown sugar (.33 cup)
- ❖ Egg (1 large)
- ❖ Vanilla sugar-free yogurt (.33 cup)
- ❖ Carrot (.75 cup)
- ❖ Banana (.5 cup)
- ❖ Vanilla extract (1 tsp.)
- ❖ Pecans (.25 cup)

Preparation Technique:

1. Place paper/foil liners in a six-cup muffin tin.
2. Mash the bananas, shred the carrot, and chop the pecans. Set them aside.
3. Combine the first five fixings (up to the line **) in a large mixing container.
4. Whisk the oil with the sugar and egg in another container. Mix in the yogurt, carrots, banana, and vanilla. Stir the oil mix into the flour mixture in a big mixing container. Fold in the pecans.
5. Scoop the batter evenly into the muffin cups.
6. Set a timer to bake at 375° Fahrenheit or 191° Celsius until muffins are lightly browned as desired (22 min.).

Carrot Cake Muffins

Servings Provided: 8

Time Required: 40 minutes

Macro Counts - Each Serving:

- Calories: 189
- Carbs: 17.3 g
- Sugar: 5.6 g
- Fiber: 3.9 g
- Chol: -0- mg
- Prot.: 3.8 g
- Sodium: 226.5 mg
- Fat Content: 13.9 g (Saturated: 8.4 g)

Ingredients Needed:

- Dry Components:
- Almond flour (1.75 cups/170 g)
- Baking soda (1 tsp.)
- Tapioca starch (.25 cup/.32 g)
- Granulated sweetener of choice - ex. Xylitol (.5 cup/15 g)
- Baking powder - gluten-free (1 tsp.)
- Nutmeg (1 tsp.)
- Cinnamon (1 tbsp.)
- Salt (1 tsp.)
- Cloves (.25 tsp.)
- Wet Components:
- Coconut oil (.33 cup/0.8 dl)
- Vanilla extract (1 tsp.)
- Banana - overripe and mashed (1 medium)
- Shredded carrots (1.5 cups/75 g)
- Flax meal (4 tbsp.) + Water (.5 cup/2.2 dl) = a flax egg for vegan OR
- *Eggs (2 large) if you are not vegan

Preparation Technique:

1. Set the oven temperature at 350° Fahrenheit or 177 ° Celsius.
2. Prepare a muffin tray with paper cups.
3. Toss each of the dry fixings into a mixing container. Thoroughly whisk to remove all of the lumps.
4. Whisk ½ cup of water with the flax meal until it becomes a "flax egg." Wait for five minutes.
5. Use your thumb to make a hole in the middle of the dry components. Mix in the flax egg, coconut oil, and vanilla extract. Combine to create a rough dough, but avoid over-mixing.
6. Mash the bananas and shred the carrots. Toss them into the mixture until just incorporated.
7. Scoop the muffin batter into the cups filling them to the tops.
8. Bake the muffins for 35 to 40 minutes.
9. Cool in the tray for ten minutes. At that time, transfer them to a rack to cool slightly before serving.

Pumpkin Raspberry Muffins - Gluten-Free

Servings Provided: 12

Time Required: 1 hour

Macro Counts - Each Serving:

- ❖ Calories: 217
- ❖ Carbs: 14.2g
- ❖ Fiber: 4.6g
- ❖ Sugar: 2.5 g
- ❖ Chol: 62 mg
- ❖ Prot.: 4.9 g
- ❖ Fat Content: 14.1 g (Saturated: 9.1 g)
- ❖ Sodium: 125.4 mg
- ❖ Net Carbs: 9.6 g

Ingredients Needed:

- ❖ Canned pumpkin puree (1 cup)
- ❖ Coconut flour (.5 cup)
- ❖ Blanched almond flour (.75 cup)
- ❖ Tapioca or arrowroot starch (3 tbsp.)
- ❖ Baking powder (1 tbsp.)
- ❖ Stevia (.5 cup)
- ❖ Salt (.25 tsp.)
- ❖ Nutmeg (1 pinch)
- ❖ Cinnamon (1 tbsp.)
- ❖ Egg whites (4/.5 cup)
- ❖ Egg yolks (4)
- ❖ Coconut oil (melted @ .5 cup)
- ❖ Vanilla extract (1.5 tsp.)
- ❖ Frozen raspberries (1.5 cups)
- ❖ Liquid stevia (10 drops)
- ❖ Needed: 12-count muffin tin

Preparation Technique:

1. Prep the oven temperature to reach 350° Fahrenheit or 177 ° Celsius.
2. Place paper liners in the muffin cups.
3. Sift or whisk the coconut flour with the almond flour, stevia, tapioca starch, baking powder, nutmeg, cinnamon, and sea salt.
4. Whisk and mix in the egg yolks, pumpkin puree, vanilla, stevia drops, and coconut oil.
5. Use another container and briskly whisk the egg whites to create stiff white peaks. Mix in the frozen raspberries and add them into the muffin batter using a spoon or spatula.
6. Scoop the batter into the cups, filling them to the top of the muffin papers.
7. Set the timer to bake for 25 minutes. Cool in the muffin tray for five minutes. At that time, arrange them on a cooling rack until ready to serve.

Chapter 4

Custard - Pudding
and Mousse

Banana & Raspberry High-Protein Mousse

Servings Provided: 1

Time Required: 5 minutes

Macro Counts - Each Serving:

- ❖ Calories: 122
- ❖ Carbs: 19.5 g
- ❖ Sugar: 9.3 g
- ❖ Fiber: 5.3 g
- ❖ Chol: -0- mg
- ❖ Prot.: 11.3 g
- ❖ Sodium: 153.8 mg
- ❖ Fat Content: 0.2 g (Saturated: 0.1 g)
- ❖ Net Carbs: 14.2

Ingredients Needed:

- ❖ Egg whites (2) or Liquid egg white (90 g)
- ❖ Stevia (1 tbsp.)
- ❖ Frozen banana (2 oz./60 g)
- ❖ Frozen raspberry (1.75 oz./45 g)

❖ Optional: Fresh berries

Preparation Technique:

1. Whisk or blend the egg whites with the stevia until they are firm (1-2 minutes). Mix in the berries and banana.
2. Once it's all pink and smooth, enjoy it in a serving dish with a garnish of fresh berries.

Eggnog Mousse

Servings Provided: 4

Time Required: 15 minutes + chill time

Macro Counts - Each Serving:

- ❖ ¾ cup serving:
- ❖ Calories: 165
- ❖ Carbs: 21 g
- ❖ Fiber: -0- g
- ❖ Sugar: 17 g
- ❖ Chol: 97 mg
- ❖ Protein: 7 g
- ❖ Sodium: 80 mg
- ❖ Fat Content: 6 g (Saturated: 4 g)
  D.E:
- ❖ Starch: 1
- ❖ Reduced-fat Milk: ½

Ingredients Needed:

- ❖ Reduced-fat eggnog (2 cups)
- ❖ Unflavored gelatin (2 tsp.)
- ❖ Ground nutmeg (0.125 tsp. + more to garnish)
- ❖ Sugar (2 tbsp.)
- ❖ Ground cinnamon (0.125 tsp.)
- ❖ Vanilla extract (.5 tsp.)
- ❖ Reduced-fat whipped topping - divided (1 cup)

Preparation Technique:

1. Use a small saucepan, and add the gelatin with the eggnog. Warm the pan using the low-temperature setting to liquefy the mixture (1 min.).

2. Mix in the cinnamon, nutmeg, and sugar - stirring until the sugar is liquified. Add the mousse mixture to a small mixing container and combine it with the vanilla. Pop it into the fridge until thickened.
3. Whisk the mixture until it's fluffy. Mix in the whipped topping (¾ cup).
4. Portion the mousse into dessert bowls and pop them into the fridge to set.
5. Garnish with the rest of the whipped topping and a sprinkle of nutmeg to your liking.

Pumpkin Pie Custard

Servings Provided: 10

Time Required: 55 minutes + chill time

Macro Counts - Each Serving:

- ❖ Topping Counts Not Included:
- ❖ Calories: 120
- ❖ Carbs: 24 g
- ❖ Sugar: 21 g
- ❖ Fiber: 2 g
- ❖ Chol: 2 mg
- ❖ Protein: 7 g
- ❖ Sodium: 151 mg
- ❖ Fat Content: -0- g (Saturated: -0- g)
  D.E:
- ❖ Starch: 1 ½

Ingredients Needed:

- ❖ Pumpkin (15 oz. can)
- ❖ Egg whites (8 large)
- ❖ Evaporated milk - fat-free (12 oz. can)
- ❖ Milk - fat-free (.5 cup)
  ****
- ❖ Ground nutmeg (.25 tsp.)
- ❖ Sugar (.75 cup)
- ❖ Ground cloves (.25 tsp.)
- ❖ Cinnamon (1 tsp.)
- ❖ Salt (.25 tsp.)
- ❖ Ground ginger (.5 tsp.)
- ❖ Optional: Sweetened whipped cream + more cinnamon
- ❖ Also Needed:
- ❖ 15x10x1-inch baking pan

❖ Ramekins/custard cups (10 @ 6 oz. each)

Preparation Technique:

1. Warm the oven to reach 350° Fahrenheit/177 ° Celsius.
2. Lightly spritz the baking pan with a cooking oil spray.
3. Arrange the ramekins in the baking tray.
4. Whisk the first four fixings (up to the **line) until smooth. Mix in the salt with the spices and sugar. Portion the custard into the custard cups.
5. Bake for 40-45 minutes. Place the pan of custard on a rack to cool.
6. Pop them into the fridge or serve within two hours.
7. Garnish the custard using a portion of whipped cream and a dusting of cinnamon.

Chapter 5

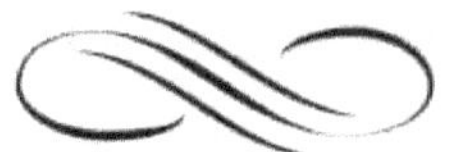

Delicious Cakes

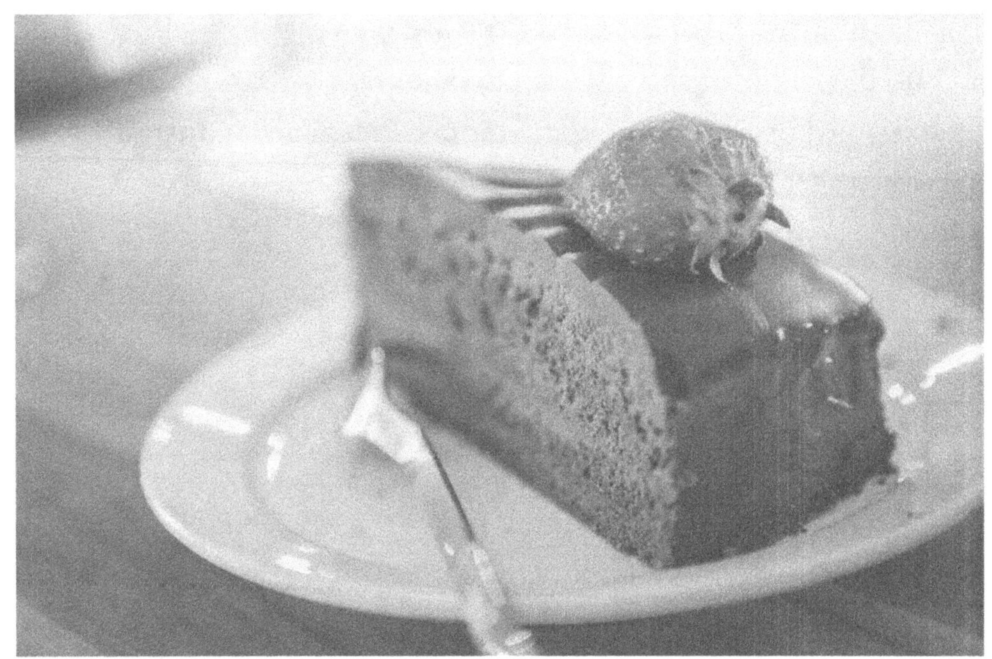

Servings Provided: 10

Time Required: 1 hour 5 minutes

Macro Counts - Each Serving:

- ❖ Calories: 138
- ❖ Carbs: 6.5 g
- ❖ Sugar: 1.8 g
- ❖ Fiber: 1.4 g
- ❖ Chol: 55.5 mg
- ❖ Protein: 3.9 g

- ❖ Sodium: mg
- ❖ Fat Content: 11.5 g (Saturated: 4.3 g)

Ingredients Needed:

- ❖ Ripe banana (.5 cup/2 small)
- ❖ Eggs (3 large)
- ❖ Coconut oil (3 tbsp.)
- ❖ Almond flour (1.5 cups)
- ❖ Xanthan gum (2 tbsp.)
- ❖ Granulated stevia (.33 cup)
- ❖ Baking powder (1.5 tsp.)
- ❖ Cinnamon (2 tsp.)
- ❖ Nutmeg (1 pinch)
- ❖ Pecans or walnuts (.5 cup - crushed)
- ❖ Also Needed: 7.5-inch loaf tin

Preparation Technique:

1. Warm the oven at 350° Fahrenheit/177 ° Celsius.
2. Cover the baking pan using a layer of parchment baking paper. Set aside.
3. Mash the bananas and mix with the eggs and melted coconut oil. Use an electric mixer to thoroughly blend until it's smooth.
4. In another mixing container, combine the almond flour with the xanthan gum, granulated stevia, nutmeg, cinnamon, and baking powder.
5. Combine the dry fixings with the wet and mix until the batter is smooth and incorporated. Fold in the crushed nuts.
6. Empty the prepared batter into the pan. Use a spatula to even the batter.
7. Set a timer to cook for 35 to 40 minutes until done.
8. Remove and cool it for 15 to 20 minutes in the tin.
9. When the loaf is cooled slightly, remove it from the tin and thoroughly cool it before slicing.

Banana Souffle

Servings Provided: 6

Time Required: 55 minutes

Macro Counts - Each Serving:

- ❖ Calories: 168
- ❖ Carbs: 21 g
- ❖ Sugar: 16 g
- ❖ Fiber: 1 g
- ❖ Chol: 151 mg
- ❖ Protein: 5 g
- ❖ Sodium: 83 mg
- ❖ Fat Content: 7 g (Saturated: 3 g)
  D.E:
- ❖ Starch: 1
- ❖ Fat: 1
- ❖ Fruit: ½

Ingredients Needed:

- ❖ Eggs - separated (4 large)
- ❖ Egg white (1 large)
- ❖ Butter (2 tbsp.)
- ❖ Ripened bananas (1 cup)
- ❖ Cornstarch (1 tbsp.)
- ❖ Grated lemon zest (.25 tsp.)
- ❖ Rum (1 tbsp.)
- ❖ Sugar (.33 cup)
- ❖ Lemon juice (1 tbsp.)
- ❖ Also Needed: 1.5-quart souffle dish

Preparation Technique:

1. Place the egg whites on the countertop for ½ hour. Coat the souffle dish with a spritz of cooking oil spray.
2. Warm a saucepan on the stovetop - set using the medium-temperature setting. Melt the butter. Mash and add the bananas, cornstarch, and sugar, mixing until blended.
3. Wait for it to boil, continually stirring. Cook and stir the mixture for one to two more minutes or until thickened. Empty the mixture into a big mixing container. Mix in the rum, lemon juice, and zest.
4. Fold in a minimal portion of the hot mix into the egg yolks and add all of the fixings back into the bowl, continually mixing. Slightly cool and set aside.
5. In another container, vigorously beat the egg whites to create "stiff" peaks.
6. Slowly mix in ¼ of the egg whites into the banana mixture. Stir in the remainder of the egg whites until combined.
7. Scoop it into the baking dish.
8. Bake at 350° Fahrenheit or 177 ° Celsius until the top is puffed and the center appears set (½ hour). Enjoy it promptly.

Chocolate & Banana Cake

Servings Provided: 12

Time Required: 40 minutes + cool time

Macro Counts - Each Serving:

- ❖ Calories: 169
- ❖ Carbs: 25 g
- ❖ Sugar: 10 g
- ❖ Fiber: 1 g
- ❖ Chol: 45 mg
- ❖ Prot.: 4 g
- ❖ Sodium: 261 mg
- ❖ Fat Content: 6 g (Saturated: 4 g)
  D.E:
- ❖ Starch: 1 ½
- ❖ Fat: 1

Ingredients Needed:

- ❖ Unchilled butter (.33 cup)
- ❖ Packed brown sugar (.33 cup)
- ❖ Vanilla extract (2 tsp.)
- ❖ Sugar substitute (equal to 0.75 cup sugar)
- ❖ Unchilled large eggs (2)
- ❖ Water (.5 cup)
- ❖ Baking cocoa (3 tbsp.)
- ❖ Nonfat dry milk powder (.5 cup)
- ❖ Bak. soda (.5 tsp.)
- ❖ A.P. flour (1.33 cups)
- ❖ Salt (.5 tsp.)
- ❖ Bak. powder (1 tsp.)
- ❖ Mashed ripe bananas (1 cup/about 2 medium)
- ❖ Confectioners' sugar

❖ Suggested: 9-inch square baking pan

Preparation Technique:

1. Set the oven temperature at 375° F/191° C.
2. Lightly spritz a baking pan using cooking oil spray.
3. Beat the butter with both types of sugar until creamy.
4. Add the vanilla and water. Mix in the eggs individually, thoroughly mixing after adding each one.
5. Whisk the flour with the baking powder, milk powder, baking soda, salt, and cocoa. Mix it in with the creamed mixture - stirring until just combined. Lastly, mix in the bananas.
6. Scoop the mixture into the pan.
7. Bake until the cake begins to pull from the pan's sides (23-28 min.).
8. Leave it in the pan and set it aside to cool thoroughly before dusting it using a bit of confectioner' sugar to serve.

Chocolate Zucchini Snack Cake

Servings Provided: 18

Time Required: 50 minutes

Macro Counts - Each Serving:

- ❖ Calories: 172
- ❖ Carbs: 29 g
- ❖ Sugar: 17 g
- ❖ Fiber: 1 g
- ❖ Chol: 33 mg
- ❖ Protein: 3 g
- ❖ Sodium: 223 mg
- ❖ Fat Content: 5 g (Saturated: 3 g)
  D.E:
- ❖ Starch: 2
- ❖ Fat: 1

Ingredients Needed:

- ❖ Unchilled butter (.33 cup)
- ❖ Eggs (2)
- ❖ Buttermilk (.5 cup)
- ❖ Sugar (1.25 cups)
- ❖ Applesauce - unsweetened (.33 cup)
- ❖ Vanilla extract (1 tsp.)
- ❖ Semisweet chocolate - melted (2 oz.)
- ❖ Bak. soda (.25 tsp.)
- ❖ A.P. flour (2.25 cups)
- ❖ Salt (1 tsp.)
- ❖ Bak. powder (1.5 tsp.)
- ❖ Shredded zucchini (2 cups)
- ❖ Confectioners' sugar (2 tsp.)
- ❖ Also Needed: 13x9-inch baking dish

Preparation Technique:

1. Use a big mixing container to cream the sugar and butter together until it crumbles (two min.).
2. Whisk and mix in the eggs. Beat in the applesauce, chocolate, buttermilk, and vanilla. Sift the baking powder with the baking soda, flour, and salt, mixing it into butter mixture just until moistened. Add in the zucchini.
3. Scoop the mixture into the baking dish coated with a spritz of baking oil spray.
4. Bake the cake at 350° Fahrenheit or 177 ° Celsius for ½ hour to 35 minutes.
5. Place it on a rack to cool and add a dusting of confectioners' sugar to serve.

Mocha Angel Cake With Chai-Spiced Cream

Servings Provided: 12

Time Required: 1 hour 50 minutes

Macro Counts - Each Serving:

- ❖ Calories: 137
- ❖ Carbs: 26.5 g
- ❖ Sugar: 17.4 g
- ❖ Fiber: 0.2 g
- ❖ Chol: -0- mg
- ❖ Prot: 4 g
- ❖ Sodium: 42.6 mg
- ❖ Fat Content: 17.4 g (Saturated: 1.4 g)
  D.E.:
- ❖ Other Carbs: 1 ½

Ingredients Needed:

- ❖ Egg whites (1.25 cups/8-10 large eggs)
- ❖ Granulated sugar (.66 or 2/3 cup)
- ❖ A.P. flour (.75 cup)
- ❖ Cocoa powder - unsweetened (.25 cup)
- ❖ Cream of tartar (1.25 tsp.)
- ❖ Powdered sugar (.5 cup)
- ❖ Crushed instant coffee crystals/Instant espresso coffee powder (1 tbsp.)
- ❖ Vanilla extract (.5 tsp.)
- ❖ Chai-Spiced Cream (1 recipe - below)
- ❖ The Cream:
- ❖ Light whipped dessert topping - frozen (½ - 8 oz. container)
- ❖ Ground cardamom (.125 tsp.)
- ❖ Cinnamon (.125 tsp.)
- ❖ Spices @ 1 pinch each:
- ❖ Ground cloves

- ❖ Nutmeg
- ❖ Ground black pepper
- ❖ Ground ginger
- ❖ Optional: Chocolate-covered coffee beans (12)
- ❖ Also Needed: 10-inch tube pan

Preparation Technique:

1. Thaw the dessert topping.
2. Place the oven rack in the bottom position. Warm the oven temperature to 350° Fahrenheit or 177° Celsius.
3. Break and place the egg whites in a holding container on the countertop for ½ hour.
4. Sift the flour, cocoa powder, powdered sugar, and espresso powder thoroughly (3 times). You need to be sure it is lump-free.
5. Adjust the baking rack to the lowest position in the oven.
6. Use an electric mixer to blend the vanilla and cream of tartar with the egg whites using the medium-speed setting until soft peaks form.
7. Slowly add the granulated sugar (2 tbsp. at a time), once again, blending until stiff peaks are formed.
8. Sift ¼ of the flour mixture over beaten egg whites, folding it in gently. Continue folding in the rest of the flour mixture using 1/3 portions. Spoon the mixture into an ungreased pan.
9. Bake the cake until the top springs back when lightly touched (30-35 min.).
10. Promptly invert the cake into the pan and wait for it to thoroughly cool. Loosen the sides of the cake from the pan and remove it
11. Prepare the cream. Put thawed light whipped dessert topping in a medium mixing container. Add the cardamom with the black pepper, ground cloves, cinnamon, nutmeg, and ginger. Toss gently to combine.
12. Scoop the cream into 12 small portions around the edge and top of the cake. Decorate each one with a coffee bean.

Orange Dream Angel Food Cake

Servings Provided: 16

Time Required: 55 minutes + cool time

Macro Counts - Each Serving:

- ❖ Calories: 130
- ❖ Carbs: 28 g
- ❖ Sugar: 22 g
- ❖ Prot.: 4 g
- ❖ Fat Content: -0- g
- ❖ Sodium: 116 mg
  D.E:
- ❖ Starch: 2

Ingredients Needed:

- ❖ Unchilled egg whites (12 large)
- ❖ Salt (.5 tsp.)
- ❖ Cream of tartar (1.5 tsp.)
- ❖ A.P. flour (1 cup)
- ❖ Sugar - divided (1.75 cups)
- ❖ Orange - Almond & vanilla extract (1 tsp. each)
- ❖ Orange zest (1 tsp.)
- ❖ Optional: Yellow & red food coloring (6 drops of each)
- ❖ Needed: Tube pan (10-inch)

Preparation Technique:

1. Separate the egg whites in a large mixing container for ½ hour to unchill. Grease the pan and place it to the side for now.
2. Sift or whisk the flour with the sugar (¾ cup). Set the container to the side.
3. Whisk the salt and cream of tartar with the vanilla and almond extracts - mixing them into the egg whites.

4. Use a mixer (medium-speed setting) to create soft peaks. Slowly mix in the rest of the sugar (2 tbsp. at a time), beating on high until stiff glossy peaks form and the sugar is liquified. Slowly mix in the flour mixture (½ cup portions).

5. Scoop ½ of the batter into the greased pan.

6. Mix in the orange zest with the food coloring, orange extract, and the rest of the batter. Scoop small portions of the orange batter over white batter. Swirl it using a toothpick.

7. Position the oven rack on it's lowest level. Bake at 375° Fahrenheit or 191° Celsius until browned (30-35 min.). Promptly invert the pan and thoroughly cool (1 hr.).

8. You may need to run a butter knife around the pan's edges and place the cake onto a serving plate.

Peanut Butter Cake

Servings Provided: 24

Time Required: 35 minutes

Macro Counts - Each Serving:

- ❖ Calories: 220
- ❖ Carbs: 31g
- ❖ Fiber: 1 g
- ❖ Sugar: 22 g
- ❖ Chol: 30 mg
- ❖ Prot.: 4 g
- ❖ Sodium: 166 mg
- ❖ Fat Content: 9 g (Saturated: 4 g)
  D.E.:
- ❖ Starch: 2
- ❖ Fat: 1 ½

Ingredients Needed:

- ❖ Creamy-style peanut butter (.5 cup)
- ❖ Butter - cubed (6 tbsp.)
- ❖ Water (1 cup)
- ❖ A.P. flour (2 cups)
- ❖ Sugar (1.5 cups)
- ❖ Buttermilk (.5 cup)
- ❖ Unsweetened applesauce (.25 cup)
- ❖ Large eggs (2 lightly beaten)
- ❖ Bak. powder (1.25 tsp.)
- ❖ Vanilla extract (1 tsp.)
- ❖ Salt (.5 tsp.)
- ❖ Bak. soda (.25 tsp.)
- ❖ The Frosting:
- ❖ Butter - cubed (.25 cup)

- ❖ Peanut butter - creamy (.25 cup)
- ❖ Vanilla extract (1 tsp.)
- ❖ Milk - fat-free (2 tbsp.)
- ❖ Confectioners' sugar (1.75 cups)
- ❖ Suggested: 15x10x1-inch baking pan

Preparation Technique:

1. Prepare a large saucepan and add the peanut butter, water, and butter - just to a boil. Immediately take the pan from the burner.
2. Mix in the buttermilk, flour, eggs, applesauce, baking powder, sugar, salt, baking soda, and vanilla. Thoroughly stir until it's creamy smooth.
3. Empty the batter into the baking pan coated with a bit of cooking oil spray.
4. Set a timer and bake at 375° Fahrenheit or 191° Celsius until they are a nice brown to your liking (15-20 min.). Wait for it to cool on the countertop for 20 minutes.
5. Melt the butter and peanut butter in a saucepan using the medium temperature setting. Stir in the milk and wait for it to boil. Immediately transfer the pan from the burner.
6. Mix in the confectioners' sugar and vanilla until it's creamy smooth.
7. Spread the mixture over the warm cake. Thoroughly cool it using a wire rack.
8. Refrigerate any leftovers for another time.

Pear Bundt Cake

Servings Provided: 16

Time Required: 55 minutes + cooling time

Macro Counts - Each Serving:

- ❖ Calories: 149
- ❖ Carbs: 28 g
- ❖ Sugar: 16 g
- ❖ Fiber: 0 g
- ❖ Chol: 12 mg
- ❖ Prot.: 2 g
- ❖ Sodium: 232 mg
- ❖ Fat Content: 3 g (Saturated: 1 g)
  D.E.:
- ❖ Starch: 2
- ❖ Fat: ½

Ingredients Needed:

- ❖ Sliced pears - reduced-sugar (15 oz. can)
- ❖ White cake mix (16.25 oz./regular size pkg.)
- ❖ Egg whites - unchilled (2 large)
- ❖ Egg- unchilled (1 large)
- ❖ Confectioners' sugar (2 tsp.)
- ❖ Pan Needed: Ten-inch fluted tube pan

Preparation Technique:

1. Drain the pears, saving the syrup.
2. Chop the pears and place them with the syrup in a big mixing container.
3. Whisk and mix the egg whites and egg with the cake mix and blend them using the low-speed setting of an electric mixer (30 sec.). Beat using the high setting for four minutes.
4. Spritz the pan with cooking oil spray and a sprinkle of flour. Add batter.
5. Bake at 350° Fahrenheit or 177 ° Celsius for 48-55 minutes.

6. Cool the cake for ten minutes before removing from the pan to a wire rack to thoroughly cool.
7. Sprinkle the cake using the sugar to serve.

Layered Cakes

Almond-Pistachio Dessert Roll-Ups

Servings Provided: 1.5 dozen

Time Required: 45 minutes

Macro Counts - Each Serving:

- ❖ Calories: 83
- ❖ Carbs: 10 g
- ❖ Sugar: 5 g
- ❖ Fiber: 1 g
- ❖ Chol: 2 mg
- ❖ Prot: 2 g
- ❖ Sodium: 50 mg
- ❖ Fat Content: 4 g (Saturated: 1 g)
  D.E:
- ❖ Starch: ½
- ❖ Fat: 1
- ❖ Fruit:

Ingredients Needed:

- ❖ Shelled pistachios, toasted (.5 cup)
- ❖ Unblanched whole almonds, toasted (.25 cup)
- ❖ Sugar (1 tbsp.)
- ❖ Unchilled butter - softened (1 tbsp.)
- ❖ Ground cinnamon (.5 tsp.)
- ❖ Phyllo dough (12 sheets @ 14x9-inch each)
- ❖ Butter-flavored cooking spray
- ❖ Honey - divided (.25 cup)

Preparation Technique:

1. Warm the oven at 325° F/163° C.

2. Toss the pistachios and almonds into a food processor. Close the top and pulse the nuts until they're finely chopped. Measure and pour in the cinnamon, sugar, and butter. Securely close the lid and pulse until chopped and blended.

3. Arrange one sheet of phyllo dough on a work surface. Spray with a portion of cooking spray.

4. Continue with the second layer. Spread the nut mixture (1/3 cup) over phyllo to within one inch of sides and drizzle with one tablespoon honey.

5. Layer with two more sheets of phyllo. Be sure to spray each layer with cooking spray.

6. Roll it up, starting from the short side. Continue using the rest of the phyllo, nut mixture, and honey.

7. Slice each roll into six pieces. Place them with the seam side down onto a greased baking sheet. Lightly spritz using a baking oil spray. Bake until it's golden (16-20 min.). Drizzle with the rest of the honey to serve.

Cream Cheese Streusel Bars

Servings Provided: 16

Time Required: 50 minutes + cool time

Macro Counts - Each Serving:

- ❖ Calories: 216
- ❖ Carbs: 28 g
- ❖ Sugar: 21 g
- ❖ Fiber: -0- g
- ❖ Chol: 40 mg
- ❖ Prot: 5 g
- ❖ Sodium: 164 mg
- ❖ Fat Content: 9 g (Saturated: 6 g)
  D.E:
- ❖ Starch: 2
- ❖ Fat: 2

Ingredients Needed:

- ❖ A.P. flour (1 cup)
- ❖ Confectioners' sugar (.75 cup)
- ❖ Baking cocoa (.25 cup)
- ❖ Salt (.125 tsp.)
- ❖ Baking soda (.125 tsp.)
- ❖ Cold butter - cubed (.5 cup)
- ❖ The Filling:
- ❖ Reduced-fat cream cheese (8 oz. pkg.)
- ❖ Condensed milk - sweetened - fat-free (14 oz. can)
- ❖ Egg - lightly beaten (1 large)
- ❖ Vanilla extract (2 tsp.)
- ❖ Needed: 8-inch square baking pan

Preparation Technique:

1. Program the oven setting 350° Fahrenheit/177 ° Celsius.
2. Sift or whisk the first five fixings. Cut in the butter until fine crumbs form (mixture will be powdery).
3. Reserve ½ cup of the mixture for the topping. Lightly press the rest of the mixture into the baking pan coated with a spritz of cooking oil spray. Bake just until set (8-10 minutes).
4. Mix the cream cheese until it's creamy. Slowly mix in the egg, vanilla, and milk, beating - just until incorporated. Dump it over the crust.
5. Set a timer and bake it for 15 minutes.
6. Sprinkle the reserved topping overfilling. Bake until filling is set (5-10 min.). Thoroughly cool on a rack. Store in the fridge.

Orange Ricotta Cake Roll

Servings Provided: 12

Time Required: 55 minutes + chill time

Macro Counts - Each Serving:

- Calories: 169
- Carbs: 17 g
- Sugar: 14 g
- Fiber: -0- g
- Chol: 94 mg
- Prot.: 7 g
- Sodium: 95 mg
- Fat Content: 9 g (Saturated: 5 g)
  D.E:
- Fat: 2
- Starch: 1

Ingredients Needed:

- Eggs @ room temperature (4 large - separated)
- Vanilla extract (1 tsp.)
- Baking cocoa (.25 cup)
- A.P. flour (2 tbsp.)
- Salt (.125 tsp.)
- Cream of tartar (.5 tsp.)
- Confectioners' sugar - sifted - divided (.66 cup)
- The Filling:
- Mascarpone cheese (3 tbsp.)
- Ricotta cheese (15 oz. container)
- Sugar (.33 cup)
- Grated orange zest (1 tbsp.)
- Kahlua - coffee liqueur (1 tbsp.)
- Vanilla extract (.5 tsp.)

- ❖ Additional confectioners' sugar
- ❖ Also Needed: 15x10x1-inch baking pan

Preparation Technique:

1. Separate and add the egg whites into a bowl. Set the oven temperature at 325° F/163° C.
2. Cover the base of a greased baking pan with a parchment paper layer, and lightly grease/oil the paper.
3. Sift the flour with the cocoa and salt - twice.
4. Whisk the egg yolks in another container until slightly thickened.
5. Slowly mix in 1/3 cup confectioners' sugar (high speed) until thickened. Beat in vanilla. Fold in the cocoa mixture.
6. Mix the cream of tartar to the egg whites. Mix using the medium setting to create soft peaks. Slowly mix in the rest of the confectioners' sugar (1 tbsp. at a time). After soft glossy peaks form, fold ¼ of the whites into the batter, and the remaining whites. Pour it into the pan.
7. Bake until the top springs back when lightly touched (9-11 min.). Cover the cake using a layer of waxed paper and cool thoroughly on a wire rack.
8. Discard the waxed paper and invert the cake onto an 18-inch-long sheet of waxed paper dusted with confectioners' sugar. Peel off the layer of parchment paper.
9. In another container, mix the cheeses and sugar until blended. Stir in the Kahlua, zested orange bits, and vanilla. Spread the mixture over the cake to within ½ inch of the edges.
10. Roll it up, beginning with a short side. Trim the ends and place them on a platter with the seam side down.
11. Pop the roll into the fridge, covered, at least one hour before serving.
12. To serve, dust with confectioners' sugar.

Pumpkin-Butterscotch Gingerbread Trifle

Servings Provided: 16

Time Required: 1.25 hours + cooling time

Macro Counts - Each Serving:

- ❖ ¾ cup servings:
- ❖ Carbohydrates: 33 g
- ❖ Calories: 220
- ❖ Sugar: 18 g
- ❖ Fiber: 1 g
- ❖ Chol: 13 mg
- ❖ Prot.: 4 g
- ❖ Sodium: 325 mg
- ❖ Fat Content: 6 g (Saturated: 3 g)
  D.E:
- ❖ Starch: 2
- ❖ Fat: 1

Ingredients Needed:

- ❖ Gingerbread cake/cookie mix (14.5 oz. pkg.)
- ❖ Cold milk - fat-free (4 cups)
- ❖ Instant butterscotch pudding mix - sugar-free (4 pkg. @1 oz. each)
- ❖ Ground cinnamon (1 tsp.)
- ❖ Pumpkin (15 oz. can)
- ❖ Ground ginger - nutmeg & allspice (.25 tsp. each)
- ❖ Frozen & thawed reduced-fat whipped topping (12 oz. carton)

Preparation Technique:

1. Prepare and bake the gingerbread per the package instructions. Cool it thoroughly.
2. Crumble the cake, reserving ¼ of a cup of crumbs.
3. Whisk the milk with the pudding mixes and spices until thickened (2 min.). Stir in the pumpkin.

4. Use a glass bowl or 3.5-quart trifle to layer ¼ of the cake crumbs, ½ of the pumpkin mixture, ¼ of the cake crumbs, and ½ of the whipped topping. Make another layer.
5. Top with the last of the crumbs (step 2) and pop it into the fridge until it's time to serve.

Tiramisu Delight

Servings Provided: 9

Time Required: 25 minutes + chill time

Macro Counts - Each Serving:

- ❖ Calories: 177
- ❖ Carbs: 25 g
- ❖ Sugar: 18 g
- ❖ Fiber: -0- g
- ❖ Sodium: 80 mg
- ❖ Fat Content: 6 g (Saturated: 4g)
- ❖ Protein: 6 g
  D.E:
- ❖ Fat: 1
- ❖ Starch: 1
- ❖ Fat-free milk: ½

Ingredients Needed:

- ❖ Ladyfinger Cookies (24)
- ❖ Heavy whipping cream (.5 cup)
- ❖ Vanilla yogurt (2 cups)
- ❖ Milk - fat-free (1 cup)
- ❖ Strong coffee/Brewed espresso - cooled (.5 cup)
- ❖ Optional:
- ❖ Fresh raspberries
- ❖ Baking cocoa
- ❖ Suggested: 8-inch square dish

Preparation Technique:

1. Beat the cream to form stiff peaks. Fold in the yogurt. Spread about ½ cup of the cream mixture into the baking dish.

2. Use a shallow dish to combine the espresso with the milk. Quickly dip half (12) of the ladyfingers into the espresso mixture. Let the excess drip off.

3. Place them in a dish in a single layer. (You can break them to pieces as needed to fit the pan.). Add half of the remaining cream mixture and dust with cocoa.

4. Repeat the layers.

5. Pop them into the fridge, covered, for at least two hours before serving with the raspberries.

Chapter 6

Cupcake Favorites

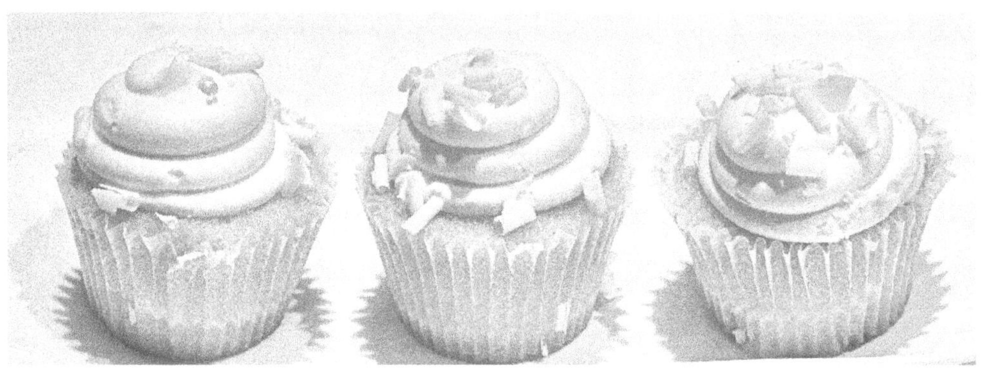

Servings Provided: 17

Time Required: 35 minutes + cool time

Macro Counts - Each Serving:

- ❖ Calories: 192
- ❖ Carbs: 33 g
- ❖ Sugar: 19 g
- ❖ Fiber: 1 g
- ❖ Chol: 22 mg
- ❖ Prot.: 3 g
- ❖ Sodium: 154 mg
- ❖ Fat Content: 5 g (Saturated: 1 g)
  D.E:
- ❖ Starch: 2
- ❖ Fat: 1

Ingredients Needed:

- ❖ Sugar (1.5 cups)
- ❖ A.P. flour (2 cups)
- ❖ Baking cocoa (.5 cup)
- ❖ Salt (.5 tsp.)
- ❖ Baking soda (1 tsp.)
- ❖ Prune baby food (.5 cup)
- ❖ Instant coffee granules (.25 cup)
- ❖ Hot water (.5 cup)
- ❖ Eggs (2)
- ❖ Canola oil (.25 cup)
- ❖ Vanilla extract (2 tsp.)
- ❖ Whipped topping - reduced-fat (1.5 cups)
- ❖ Additional baking cocoa

Preparation Technique:

1. Place paper liners in the muffin cups.
2. Sift or whisk the flour with baking soda, sugar, cocoa, and salt.
3. Dissolve the coffee in hot water. Set aside.
4. Whisk the eggs with the oil, vanilla, baby food, and coffee mixture. Gradually stir into the dry fixings - just until moistened. Fill the cups 2/3 full.
5. Bake at 350° Fahrenheit or 177 ° Celsius until a toothpick comes out clean (18-20 min.).
6. Cool them for ten minutes. Then remove them from the pans to the countertop on racks to thoroughly cool.
7. Ice the cupcakes with whipped topping and a sprinkle of cocoa right before serving. Refrigerate the leftovers for later.

Chocolate-Coconut Angel Cupcakes

Servings Provided: 1.5 dozen

Time Required: 50 minutes + cooling time

Macro Counts - Each Serving:

- ❖ Calories: 110
- ❖ Carbs: 22 g
- ❖ Sugar: 17 g
- ❖ Fiber: 1 g
- ❖ Chol: -0- mg
- ❖ Prot.: 2 g
- ❖ Sodium: 78 mg
- ❖ Fat Content: 2 g (Saturated: 2 g)
  D.E:
- ❖ Starch: 1 ½

Ingredients Needed:

- ❖ Unchilled egg whites (6 large)
- ❖ A.P. flour (.66 or 2/3 cup)
- ❖ Baking cocoa (.25 cup)
- ❖ Sugar - divided (1.33 cups)
- ❖ Baking powder (.5 tsp.)
- ❖ Almond extract (1 tsp.)
- ❖ Cream of tartar (.5 tsp.)
- ❖ Sweetened shredded coconut (1 cup)
- ❖ Salt (.25 tsp.)
- ❖ Confectioners' sugar - optional
- ❖ Muffin tin and 18 cupcake liners

Preparation Technique:

1. Break and add the egg whites into a large mixing container.
2. Set the oven temperature at 350° F/177 ° C.

3. Whisk or sift the flour with the baking powder, cocoa, and one cup of sugar twice.

4. Mix in the cream of tartar, almond extract, and salt to the egg whites. Use the mixer (medium-speed setting) to create soft peaks.

5. Slowly mix in the rest of the sugar (one tablespoon at a time) using high speed to combine them (beating after adding each one) until sugar is liquified.

6. Continue beating to form stiff glossy peaks. Slowly fold in the flour mixture (½ cup at a time). Gently fold in coconut.

7. Fill the cups 2/3 full. Bake until the top appears dry (30-35 min.).

8. Cool them in the pans for about ten minutes before transferring the cupcakes onto wire racks to cool the rest of the way. Sprinkle them using a bit of confectioner' sugar as desired.

Chocolate Macaroon Cupcakes

Servings Provided: 1.5 dozen

Time Required: 50 minutes + cool time

Macro Counts - Each Serving:

- ❖ Calories: 126
- ❖ Carbs: 24 g
- ❖ Sugar: 16 g
- ❖ Fiber: 1 g
- ❖ Chol: 14 mg
- ❖ Prot.: 4 g
- ❖ Sodium: 85 mg
- ❖ Fat Content: 2 g (Saturated: 1 g)
  D.E:
- ❖ Starch: 1 ½

Ingredients Needed:

- ❖ Egg whites (2 large)
- ❖ Unchilled egg (1 large)
- ❖ Vanilla extract (1 tsp.)
- ❖ Unsweetened applesauce (.33 cup)
  ****
- ❖ A.P. flour (1.25 cups)
- ❖ Baking cocoa (.33 cup)
- ❖ Sugar (1 cup)
- ❖ Baking soda (.5 tsp.)
- ❖ Buttermilk (.75 cup)
- ❖ The Filling:
- ❖ Ricotta cheese - reduced-fat (1 cup)
- ❖ Sugar (.25 cup)
- ❖ Egg white (1 large)
- ❖ Sweetened shredded coconut (.33 cup)

❖ Coconut or almond extract (.5 tsp.)

❖ Confectioners' sugar

Preparation Technique:

1. Warm the oven to reach 350° Fahrenheit/177 ° Celsius.
2. Coat 18 muffin cups with cooking spray.
3. Beat the first four ingredients (up to the line **) until well blended.
4. In another mixing container, whisk the flour, cocoa, baking soda, and sugar. Slowly beat into egg mixture alternately with the buttermilk.
5. Prepare the filling by beating the ricotta cheese with the egg white and sugar until it's incorporated. Mix in the coconut and extract.
6. Fill prepared cups with half of the batter. Drop the filling by tablespoonfuls into the center of each cupcake and cover with the remainder of the batter.
7. Bake them until nicely browned (27-33 min.).
8. Let them cool for ten minutes before transferring them to wire racks to finish cooling.
9. Serve with a dusting of confectioners' sugar.

Lemon Meringue Cupcakes

Servings Provided: 2 dozen

Time Required: 55 minutes + cool time

Macro Counts - Each Serving:

- ❖ Calories: 153
- ❖ Carbs: 25g
- ❖ Sugar: 16g
- ❖ Fiber: -0- g
- ❖ Sodium: 176 mg
- ❖ Chol: 28 mg
- ❖ Fat Content: 5 g (Saturated: 1 g)
- ❖ Protein: 2 g
  D.E:
- ❖ Starch: 1 ½
- ❖ Fat: 1 ½

Ingredients Needed:

- ❖ Lemon cake mix (regular size pkg.)
- ❖ Water (1-1/3 cups)
- ❖ Lemon creme pie filling (1 cup)
- ❖ Canola oil (1/3 cup)
- ❖ Unchilled eggs (3 large)
- ❖ Grated lemon zest (1 tbsp.)
- ❖ The Meringue:
- ❖ Unchilled egg whites (3 large)
- ❖ Sugar (.5 cup)
- ❖ Cream of tartar (.5 tsp.)

Preparation Technique:

1. Mix the cake mix with the oil, water, lemon zest, and eggs. Beat on low speed for ½ minute. Adjust the setting to medium for two minutes.

2. Fill 24 paper-lined muffin cups until they are approximately 2/3 of the way to full.

3. Bake at 350° Fahrenheit/177 ° Celsius until they are a nice brown (18-22 min.).

4. Snip a small hole in the corner of a plastic bag or use a pastry injector and insert a tiny tip. Fill it with the pie filling. Push the tip/end into the top of each cupcake to fill.

5. Whisk the egg whites with the cream of tartar using the medium-speed setting to create soft peaks.

6. Slowly mix in the sugar (1 tbsp. @ a time). Mix using the high-speed setting until stiff glossy peaks are formed, and the sugar is liquified. Pipe it over the tops of cupcakes.

7. Bake at 400° Fahrenheit/204° Celsius until the meringue is lightly browned (5-8 min.).

8. Cool the cupcakes for ten minutes in the pans. Then, move them to wire racks to cool thoroughly.

9. Keep the container in the fridge to enjoy as desired.

Chapter 7

Pie & Cheesecake Favorites

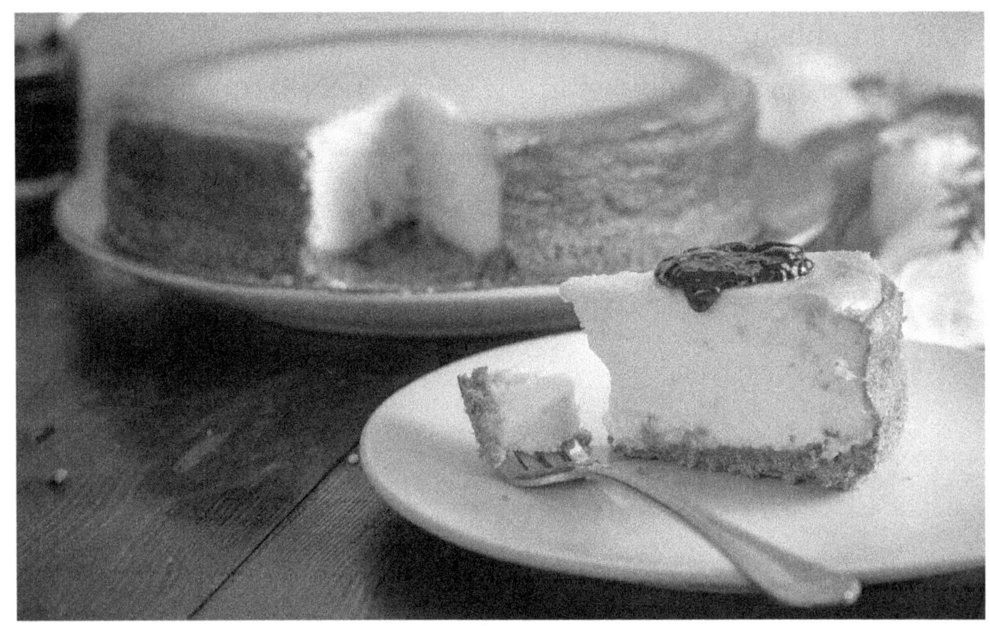

Pie Choices

Deconstructed Raspberry Pie

Servings Provided: 4

Time Required: 20 minutes

Macro Counts - Each Serving:

- ❖ Calories: 153
- ❖ Carbs: 20 g
- ❖ Sugar: 10 g
- ❖ Fiber: 6 g
- ❖ Chol: 18 mg

- ❖ Prot.: 2 g
- ❖ Sodium: 109 mg
- ❖ Fat Content: 8 g (Saturated: 4 g)

  D.E.:

- ❖ Starch: ½
- ❖ Fat: 1 ½
- ❖ Fruit: 1

Ingredients Needed:

- ❖ Fresh raspberries (2-2/3 cups)
- ❖ Melted butter (2 tbsp.)
- ❖ Sugar (2 tsp.)
- ❖ Graham cracker crumbs (.5 cup)
- ❖ Whipped cream in a can (4 tbsp.)
- ❖ Baking cocoa (.25 tsp.)
- ❖ Also Needed: 8x6-in. rectangle baking dish

Preparation Technique:

- ❖ Toss the sugar with the raspberries and set aside for now.
- ❖ Use a separate mixing container to combine the butter with the cracker crumbs. Press the mixture into the ungreased baking sheet.
- ❖ Bake at 350° Fahrenheit/177 ° Celsius until they are browned to your liking (5-6 min.). Cool them thoroughly on a wire rack before breaking them into large chunks.
- ❖ Portion ½ of the graham cracker pieces into four dessert dishes; top with raspberries (1/3 cup).
- ❖ Continue the layers, topping each one with one tablespoon of whipped cream and a sprinkle of cocoa.

Key Lime Pie

Servings Provided: 8

Time Required: 20 minutes + chill time

Macro Counts - Each Serving:

- ❖ Calories: 194
- ❖ Carbs: 33 g
- ❖ Sugar: 18 g
- ❖ Chol: 2 mg
- ❖ Prot.: 3 g
- ❖ Sodium: 159 mg
- ❖ Fat Content: 3 g (Saturated: 1 g)

  D.E:
- ❖ Starch: 2
- ❖ Fat: ½

Ingredients Needed:

- ❖ Boiling water (.25 cup)
- ❖ Sugar-free lime gelatin (0.3 oz. pkg.)
- ❖ Key lime yogurt (2 cartons @ 6 oz. each)
- ❖ Frozen & thawed fat-free whipped topping (8 oz. carton)
- ❖ Graham cracker crust - reduced-fat (8-inch)

Preparation Technique:

1. Prepare a big mixing container and add boiling water to the gelatin. Whisk it for two minutes until it is liquified.
2. Whisk in the yogurt and gently fold in the whipped topping. Dump it into the crust.
3. Pop it into the fridge with a cover until it's set (2 hrs.).

No-Bake Apple Pie

Servings Provided: 8

Time Required: 20 minutes + chill time

Macro Counts - Each Serving:

- ❖ Calories: 202
- ❖ Carbs: 30 g
- ❖ Sugar: 17 g
- ❖ Fiber: 2 g
- ❖ Chol: -0- mg
- ❖ Protein: 3 g
- ❖ Fat Content: 8 g (Saturated: 1 g)
- ❖ Sodium: 152 mg
  D.E:
- ❖ Starch: 1
- ❖ Fat: 1 ½
- ❖ Fruit: 1

Ingredients Needed:

- ❖ Ground cinnamon (.5 tsp.)
- ❖ S.F. lemon gelatin (0.3 oz. pkg.)
- ❖ Ground nutmeg (.25 tsp.)
- ❖ Water - divided (.1.75 cups)
- ❖ Tart apples (5 medium - peeled and sliced)
- ❖ S. F. - cook-&-serve vanilla pudding mix (0.8 oz. pkg.)
- ❖ Chopped nuts (.5 cup)
- ❖ Graham cracker crust - reduced-fat (6 oz.)
- ❖ Optional: Whipped topping

Preparation Technique:

1. Combine the gelatin with the nutmeg, cinnamon, and 1.5 cups water. Add the apples into a large saucepan. Wait for it to boil. Adjust the temperature setting to simmer, covered, until apples are tender (5 min.).
2. Whisk the pudding mix and the rest of the water. Stir it into the apple mixture. Cook until thickened, occasionally stirring (1 min.).
3. Remove the pan and mix in the nuts. Add it to the prepared crust.
4. Refrigerate at least two hours before serving with whipped topping or as desired.

Ribbon Pudding Pie

Servings Provided: 8

Time Required: 20 minutes + chill time

Macro Counts - Each Serving:

- Calories: 184
- Carbs: 32 g
- Fiber: 1 g
- Sugar: 13 g
- Chol: 2 mg
- Protein: 6 g
- Sodium: 427 mg
- Fat Content: 3 g (Saturated: 1 g)
  D.E:
- Starch: 2
- Fat: 1

Ingredients Needed:

- Cold fat-free milk - divided (4 cups)
- Sugar-free instant vanilla pudding mix (1 oz. pkg.)
- Reduced-fat graham cracker crust (6 oz.)
- S.F. instant butterscotch pudding mix (1 oz. pkg.)
- S.F. instant chocolate pudding mix (1.4 oz. pkg.)
  Optional:
- Whipped topping
- Finely chopped pecans

Preparation Technique:

1. Whisk the milk (1.33 cups) and vanilla pudding mix for two minutes. Spread into crust.
2. In a separate mixing container, whisk another 1.33 cups of milk with the butterscotch pudding mix for two minutes. Carefully spoon over the vanilla layer, spreading evenly.

3. Use another container to whisk the rest of the milk (1.33 cups) and chocolate pudding. Mix for two minutes. Carefully spread over the top.

4. Refrigerate until set, at least ½ hour.

5. Top it off using whipped topping and pecans to your liking.

Root Beer Float Pie

Servings Provided: 8

Time Required: 15 minutes + chill time

Macro Counts - Each Serving:

- ❖ Calories: 185
- ❖ Carbs: 27 g
- ❖ Sugar: 14 g
- ❖ Prot.: 1 g
- ❖ Sodium: 275 mg
- ❖ Fat Content: 8 g (Saturated: 4 g)
  D.E:
- ❖ Starch: 2
- ❖ Fat: 1

Ingredients Needed:

- ❖ Reduced-fat whipped topping -frozen & thawed - divided (8 oz. carton)
- ❖ Diet root beer - cold (.75 cup)
- ❖ Fat-free milk (.5 cup)
- ❖ Instant vanilla pudding mix - sugar-free (1 oz. pkg.)
- ❖ Graham cracker crust (9-inch crust/about 6 oz.)
- ❖ Optional: Maraschino cherries

Preparation Technique:

1. Set aside and refrigerate ½ cup whipped topping for garnish.
2. Whisk the milk with the root beer and pudding to mix for two minutes.
3. Mix in ½ of the remaining whipped topping.
4. Spread the remainder of whipped topping over the pie. Freeze overnight or at least eight hours.
5. Scoop the reserved whipped topping over each serving and garnish using a maraschino cherry if desired.
6. Note: It's also delicious from the freezer!

Sweedish Apple Pie

Servings Provided: 8

Time Required: 40 minutes

Macro Counts - Each Serving:

- ❖ Calories: 174
- ❖ Carbs: 25 g
- ❖ Sugar: 16 g
- ❖ Fiber: 2 g
- ❖ Chol: 26 mg
- ❖ Protein: 5 g
- ❖ Sodium: 207 mg
- ❖ Fat Content: 7 g (Saturated: 1 g)
  D.E:
- ❖ Starch: 1 ½
- ❖ Fat: 1

Ingredients Needed:

- ❖ Tart apples - chopped (2 medium)
- ❖ Whole wheat flour (.25 cup)
- ❖ Salt (.5 tsp.)
- ❖ Baking powder (1 tsp.)
- ❖ A.P. flour (.25 cup)
- ❖ Sugar (.5 cup)
- ❖ Ground cinnamon (.5 tsp.)
- ❖ Egg (1 large)
- ❖ Vanilla extract (.25 tsp.)
- ❖ Chopped - toasted pecans or walnuts (.75 cup)
- ❖ Optional: Confectioners' sugar
- ❖ Also Needed: 9-inch pie plate

Preparation Technique:

1. Warm the oven at 350° Fahrenheit or 177 ° Celsius.
2. Sift each type of flour with salt, sugar, cinnamon, and baking powder.
3. Beat the egg with the vanilla. Mix them into the dry components - just until moistened. Fold in walnuts and apples.
4. Pour it into the pie plate coated with a spritz of baking oil spray.
5. Bake them for 25-30 minutes.
6. Dust it using confectioners' sugar as desired and serve warm.

Cheesecake Choices

Berry Topped Cheesecake

Servings Provided: 12

Time Required: 4 hours 55 minutes

Macro Counts - Each Serving:

- ❖ Calories: 176
- ❖ Carbs: 14 g
- ❖ Sugar: 7 g
- ❖ Fiber: 1 g
- ❖ Chol: 28 mg
- ❖ Protein: 6 g
- ❖ Sodium: 236 mg
- ❖ Fat Content: 11 g (Saturated: 7 g)
  D.E.:
- ❖ Fat: 2
- ❖ Other Carbohydrate: 1

Ingredients Needed:

- ❖ Small pretzel twists (1.5 cups/2 oz.)
- ❖ Sliced almonds - toasted (2 tbsp.)
- ❖ Melted butter (3 tbsp.)
- ❖ Water (.33 cup)
- ❖ Unflavored gelatin (1 envelope)
- ❖ Unchilled reduced-fat cream cheese (12 oz.)
- ❖ R.F. sour cream (8 oz.)
- ❖ Confectioners' sugar (.25 cup)
- ❖ Almond extract (.5 tsp.)
- ❖ Frozen - Light whipped dessert topping - thawed (4 oz.)
- ❖ Fresh strawberries - divided (1 cup)
- ❖ Fresh blackberries or blueberries - divided (1 cup)

Preparation Technique:

1. Quarter and slice the berries into halves.
2. Toss the almonds and pretzels into a food processor.
3. Place the lid on it and pulse them until finely crushed.
4. Add butter and replace the top, and pulse the mixture thoroughly to combine.
5. Press the pretzel mixture into the bottom of an eight or nine-inch springform pan.
6. Bake until lightly browned (8 to 10 min.). Cool on a wire rack.
7. Pour the water into a saucepan. Add the gelatin (don't stir). Let it soften for about five minutes.
8. Cook and stir using the low-temperature setting until the gelatin liquefies. Let it cool slightly.
9. Use an electric mixer - using the medium setting - to combine the sour cream, cream cheese, almond extract, and confectioners' sugar. Add the gelatin mixture and beat until combined. Mix in the whipped topping.
10. Spread ½ of the filling over the cooled crust, adding ½ of the strawberries blackberries.
11. Scoop and add the remainder of the cream cheese mixture over the berries.
12. Use a layer of foil or plastic to cover the cake.
13. Chill it until set (for 4-24 hrs.).
14. Loosen the cake when removing it from the pan using a sharp knife around the edges.
15. Pop away the sides of the pan and slice the cheesecake into wedges.
16. Garnish each portion with the rest of the berries as desired.

Chocolate Mini Cheesecakes

Servings Provided: 12

Time Required: 4 hours 45 minutes

Macro Counts - Each Serving:

- ❖ Calories: 156
- ❖ Carbs: 18.9 g
- ❖ Fiber: 0.7 g
- ❖ Sugar: 15 g
- ❖ Chol: 17.3 mg
- ❖ Protein: 4.4 g
- ❖ Sodium: 147.4 mg
- ❖ Fat Content: 7.6 g (Saturated: 4.5 g)
  D.E.:
- ❖ Other Carbohydrate: 1
- ❖ Fat: 1 ½

Ingredients Needed:

- ❖ Reduced-fat vanilla wafers (12)
- ❖ R.F Unchilled cream cheese (8 oz. pkg.)
- ❖ Unchilled fat-free cream cheese (½ of an 8 oz.pkg.)
- ❖ Bittersweet/semisweet chocolate - melted & cooled (3 oz.)
- ❖ Sugar (.5 cup)
- ❖ Nonfat milk (.25 cup)
- ❖ Vanilla extract (1.5 tsp.)
- ❖ Egg white - lightly beaten (1 large)
- ❖ Dried cherries or dried apricots (.25 cup)
- ❖ Chocolate curls and/or small whole or sliced strawberries (1 oz.)
- ❖ Requested: Twelve 2.5-inch muffin cups

Preparation Technique:

1. Warm the oven to 350° Fahrenheit or 177 ° Celsius.

2. Line the cups with foil or paper bake cups. Place one wafer into each cup.

3. Beat both types of cream cheese in a mixing container using an electric mixer (medium-speed setting for ½ minute).

4. Blend in the sugar, chocolate, milk, and vanilla until thoroughly incorporated. Stir in the egg white. Finely chop and add the dried cherries/apricots. Scoop the filling into the prepared cups (3/4 full).

5. Bake until set (20 min.). Let them cool in the pan for five minutes.

6. Transfer the cheesecakes from the pan. Cool on a wire rack for about one hour.

7. Place a layer of foil or plastic wrap over the cake. Let it chill for three hours or as long as 24 hours.

8. If you like, garnish with chocolate curls or strawberries before serving.

Chocolate Swirled Cheesecake

Servings Provided: 12

Time Required: 70 minutes + chill time

Macro Counts - Each Serving:

- ❖ Calories: 187
- ❖ Carbs: 17 g
- ❖ Sugar: 14 g
- ❖ Fiber: 1 g
- ❖ Chol: 46 mg
- ❖ Prot.: 8 g
- ❖ Sodium: 378 mg
- ❖ Fat Content: 8 g (Saturated: 5 g)
  D.E:
- ❖ Starch: 1 ½
- ❖ Fat: ½
- ❖ Lean Meat: 1

Ingredients Needed:

- ❖ 2% cottage cheese (2 cups)
- ❖ Crushed chocolate wafers (1 cup/about 16 wafers)
- ❖ Reduced-fat cream cheese, cubed (8 oz. pkg.)
- ❖ Sugar (.5 cup)
- ❖ Salt (1 dash)
- ❖ Vanilla extract (1 tbsp.)
- ❖ Eggs (2 large)
- ❖ Egg white (1 large)
- ❖ Bittersweet chocolate (2 oz.)
- ❖ Optional: Fresh raspberries
- ❖ Also Needed:
- ❖ 9-inch springform pan & baking tray
- ❖ Foil (2 sheets @ 18-inches square)

Preparation Technique:

1. Line a strainer with one coffee filter or four layers of cheesecloth. Place it over a bowl. Add the cottage cheese into the strainer, refrigerate, and cover for one hour.
2. Place the springform pan over the doubled foil and wrap foil securely around the pan.
3. Spritz the inside of the pan with cooking oil spray. Press crushed wafers over the bottom and one inch up its sides.
4. Set the oven to 350° Fahrenheit or 177 ° Celsius.
5. Pulse the drained cottage cheese in a food processor until it is creamy. Measure and mix in the salt, cream cheese, and sugar, processing until blended.
6. Empty the mixture into a mixing container and whisk in the vanilla, eggs, and egg white. Add one cup of batter into a small dish and fold in the melted chocolate.
7. Empty the plain batter into the crust. Then, drop chocolate batter by spoonfuls over the plain batter. Swirl the batter with a skewer or knife. Arrange the springform pan into a larger baking pan; add one inch of boiling water to a larger pan.
8. Set a timer and bake until the center is just set (40 min.).
9. Turn off the heat in the oven and slightly open the door. Cool the cheesecake in the oven for ½ hour.
10. Transfer the springform pan from the water bath. Remove the foil. Loosen sides of cheesecake with a knife; cool on a wire rack for ½ hour. Once it's thoroughly cooled, cover and pop it into the fridge overnight.
11. Remove the rim from the pan and top with raspberries.

Chocolate-Topped Strawberry Cheesecake

Servings Provided: 12

Time Required: 45 minutes + cooling times

Macro Counts - Each Serving:

- ❖ Calories: 244
- ❖ Carbs: 29 g
- ❖ Sugar: 17 g
- ❖ Fiber: 2 g
- ❖ Chol: 16 mg
- ❖ Protein: 10 g
- ❖ Sodium: 463 mg
- ❖ Fat Content: 8 g (Saturated: 5 g)
  D.E.:
- ❖ Starch: 2
- ❖ Fat: 1 ½

Ingredients Needed:

- ❖ Chocolate graham cracker crumbs (1.25 cups/8-9 crackers)
- ❖ Melted butter (.25 cup)
- ❖ Unflavored gelatin (2 envelopes)
- ❖ Cold-water (.5 cup)
- ❖ Fresh/frozen - unsweetened strawberries - thawed (16 oz.)
- ❖ F.F. cream cheese - cubed (2 pkg. @ 8 ounces of each)
- ❖ Cottage cheese - fat-free (1 cup)
- ❖ Sugar substitute (equal to .75 cup sugar)
- ❖ Reduced-fat whipped topping - frozen & thawed - divided (8 oz. carton)
- ❖ Chocolate ice cream topping (.5 cup)
- ❖ Quartered fresh strawberries (1 cup)
- ❖ Also Needed: 9-inch springform pan

Preparation Technique:

1. Warm the oven to 350° Fahrenheit or 177° Celsius.
2. Combine the butter with the cracker crumbs. Push the crust mixture into the bottom and one inch up the sides of the baking pan coated with cooking spray.
3. Put the pan on a baking tray to bake until set (ten minutes). Thoroughly cool it on a wire rack.
4. Add the gelatin into cold water in a saucepan. Wait for about one minute. Warm it using the low-temperature setting, stirring until the gelatin is completely liquified. Remove the pan from the hot burner.
5. Remove the strawberry hulls and puree the berries in a food processor. Pour it into a mixing container and combine the cottage cheese with the cream cheese and sugar substitute into the food processor, processing until smooth. While processing, gradually add in the gelatin mixture.
6. Mix in the pureed strawberries and process until thoroughly mixed.
7. Transfer the berries into a large mixing container and fold in two cups whipped topping. Scoop it into the crust.
8. Place a layer over it and pop it into the fridge until set (two to three hrs.)
9. Use a butter knife to loosen the sides of the cheesecake and remove the rim.
10. Garnish the cake using the chocolate topping, the rest of the whipped topping, and the deliciously quartered strawberries.

Ginger-Pineapple Mini Cheesecakes

Servings Provided: 12

Time Required: 1 hour 50 minutes

Macro Counts - Each Serving:

- Calories: 124
- Carbs: 15.4 g
- Sugar: 10.7 g
- Fiber: 0.2 g
- Chol: 14 mg
- Sodium: 143.4 mg
- Fat Content: 5.1 g (Saturated: 2.4 g)
  D.E.:
- Starch: 1
- Fat: 1

Ingredients Needed:

- Nonstick cooking spray
- Gingersnap cookies, such as Nabisco® brand (15 @ 2-inches each)
- Reduced-fat cream cheese - ex. - Neufchâtel (8 oz. pkg.)
- Pineapple F.F. Greek yogurt (6 oz. container)
- Sugar substitute (2 tbsp.)**
- A.P. flour (1 tbsp.)
- Vanilla (1 tsp.)
- Ground ginger (.75 tsp.)
- Refrigerated or frozen egg product, thawed (6 tbsp.)
- Crushed pineapple - juice pack (8 oz. can)
- Finely chopped, crystallized ginger (2 tbsp.)
- Also Needed: 12-count muffin tin

Preparation Technique:

1. Preheat the oven to 350° Fahrenheit/177 ° Celsius. Drain the pineapple.

2. Line the cups with paper liners. Spray the paper bake cups using a spritz of cooking spray.
3. Add one gingersnap cookie into the bottom of each of the cups.
4. Finely crush the final three gingersnap cookies and set aside.
5. Blend the cream cheese with an electric mixer using the medium-speed setting until smooth.
6. Add the yogurt, sugar, flour, vanilla, and ground ginger, beating until combined.
7. Mix in the egg, drained pineapple, and one tablespoon of the crystallized ginger.
8. Portion the batter between the prepared bake cups. Sprinkle the last tablespoon of crystallized ginger and the reserved crushed gingersnaps over the batter in each of the cups.
9. Bake them for about 15 minutes until cheesecakes appear set. Cool in the muffin cups for 20 minutes.
10. Remove cheesecakes from the cups and cool thoroughly using a wire rack. Cover and chill them for one to four hours.
11. To serve, remove each of the cheesecakes from the paper bake cups to serve.
12. Note** The substitute should be equivalent to two tablespoons of sugar.

Lemon Cheesecake Bites

Servings Provided: 25

Time Required: 9 hours 35 minutes

Macro Counts - Each Serving:

- Calories: 142
- Carbs: 14.8g
- Fiber: 0.2 g
- Sugar: 10.4 g
- Chol: 40.7 mg
- Prot.: 4.8 g
- Sodium: 244.4 mg
- Fat Content: 7.2 g (Saturated: 3.8 g)
  D.E.:
- Fat: 1 ½
- Other Carbohydrate: ½

Ingredients Needed:

- Graham crackers (1 cup)
- Sugar (1 cup)
- Butter (3 tbsp.)
- Milk - fat-free (1 cup)
- F.F & sugar-free lemon instant pudding mix (1 cup/4-serving-size pkg.)
- Unchilled reduced-fat cream cheese - Neufchâtel (2 - 8 oz. packs)
- F.F. cream cheese - softened (8 oz. pkg.)
- Plain fat-free Greek yogurt (.25 cup)
- Salt (.25 tsp.)
- Eggs (3)
- Lemon peel (2 tbsp.)
- Lemon juice (2 tbsp.)
- White baking pieces (2 tbsp.)
- Shortening (.5 tsp.)

- ❖ Chopped pistachio nuts (2 tbsp.)
- ❖ Also Needed: 9x9x2-inch baking pan

Preparation Technique:

1. Set the oven temperature to 325° F/163° C.
2. Cover the baking tray using a layer of foil, making sure to also cover the pan's edges.
3. Finely crush the crackers and shred the lemon peel. Melt the butter.
4. Combine the crushed crackers, ¼ cup of the sugar, and the butter. Evenly push it into the prepared pan. Bake for ten minutes, then cool on a wire rack.
5. Whisk the milk with the pudding mix until smooth and set aside.
6. Beat Neufchatel cheese with the cream cheese using an electric mixer (medium-high speed setting) for ½ minute.
7. Mix in the rest of the sugar (¾ cup) with the yogurt, salt, and pudding mixture. Beat until combined.
8. Break in the eggs, mixing after each addition. Mix in one tablespoon of the lemon peel and the lemon juice until incorporated. Scoop the batter over the cooled crust.
9. Bake until a one-inch area around the outside edges appears set when gently shaken (1-1 ¼ hrs.).
10. Thoroughly cool it in the pan on a rack. Cover the cheesecake using a plastic wrap, making sure the plastic wrap touches the surface of the cheesecake to avoid condensation. Chill for a minimum of eight hours or up to one day.
11. Toss the white baking pieces and shortening into a microwave-safe bowl and melt (high @ 100% power) for 10 seconds to one minute. Stir it every 20 seconds.
12. Sprinkle it over the cheesecake with chopped pistachios.
13. Lift the cake from the pan and slice into squares.
14. Garnish the cheesecake using the rest of the lemon peel (1 tbsp.). Serve as desired.

No-Bake Cheesecake with Gingersnap Crust & Mango Puree

Servings Provided: 12

Time Required: 3 hours 35 minutes

Macro Counts - Each Serving:

- ❖ Calories: 202
- ❖ Carbs: 18.9 g
- ❖ Fiber: 0.5 g
- ❖ Sugar: 13.3 g
- ❖ Chol: 35.6 mg
- ❖ Protein: 4.6 g
- ❖ Sodium: 206.1 mg
- ❖ Fat Content: 12.4 g (Saturated: 6.9 g)
  D.E.:
- ❖ Starch: 1
- ❖ Fat: 2 ½

Ingredients Needed:

- ❖ Cooking oil spray (as needed)
- ❖ Gingersnaps (15 crumbled)
- ❖ Melted butter (3 tbsp.)
- ❖ Sugar (2 tbsp. + .33 cup)
- ❖ Unflavored gelatin (1 envelope)
- ❖ Boiling water (1 cup)
- ❖ Unchilled R.F. cream cheese - Neufchatel (2 - 8 oz. pkg.)
- ❖ Vanilla (1 tsp.)
- ❖ Lime juice (1 tbsp.)
- ❖ Medium ripened mango (1)
- ❖ Suggested: 9-inch pie plate/8-inch springform pan

Preparation Technique:

1. Lightly coat the baking container with cooking spray; set aside.

2. Finely grind the gingersnaps in a food processor. Melt and pour in the butter with two tablespoons of sugar while the mixer is running. Process the mixture until the crumbs are moistened.

3. Empty the mixture into the prepared pan, pushing it over the bottom and one inch up the baking pan's sides.

4. Whisk the gelatin with the sugar (1/3 cup). Pour in boiling water, stirring until the gelatin is liquified (5 min.).

5. Combine the vanilla with the cream cheese using the medium-speed setting of an electric mixer. Slowly mix in the gelatin mixture. Empty the mixture into the crust.

6. Peel, remove the seeds, and chop the mango; toss it into a food processor with the lime juice. Place a lid on the blender and mix until it's a smooth puree. Push the mango puree through a fine-mesh sieve and discard solids.

7. Drizzle three tablespoons of the mango puree over the cheesecake filling. Swirl it with a knife to create a marbled effect. Place a layer of foil over the cake and pop it into the fridge to chill. Add the remaining mango puree and chill for another three hours or until the cheesecake is firm.

8. To serve, discard the pan's sides and slice cheesecake into wedges.

9. Serve the remaining mango puree with cheesecake wedges or any way you desire.

No-Bake Pumpkin Swirl Cheesecake

Servings Provided: 12

Time Required: 8 hours 35 minutes

Macro Counts - Each Serving:

- ❖ Calories: 148
- ❖ Carbs: 12.2 g
- ❖ Fiber: 1.3 g
- ❖ Sugar: 2.6 g
- ❖ Chol: 22.7 mg
- ❖ Protein: 8.9 g
- ❖ Sodium: 330.9 mg
- ❖ Fat Content: 7.4 g (Saturated: 4.5 g)
  D.E.:
- ❖ Fat: 1 ½
- ❖ Other Carbs: 1 ½

Ingredients Needed:

- ❖ Graham crackers (.75 cup)
- ❖ Butter (2 tbsp.)
- ❖ Cream cheese -reduced-fat - Neufchâtel (8 oz. pkg.)
- ❖ Sugar (.5 cup)
- ❖ Milk - fat-free (.5 cup)
- ❖ Grated orange peel (.5 tsp.)
- ❖ Vanilla (2 tsp.)
- ❖ F.F cream cheese (2 @ 8 oz. pkg.)
- ❖ Pumpkin (15 oz. can)
- ❖ Pumpkin pie spice (1 tsp.)
- ❖ Orange juice (.25 cup)
- ❖ Unflavored gelatin (.25 oz. envelope)
- ❖ Also Needed: 8-inch springform baking pan

Preparation Technique:

1. First, melt the butter. Finely crush and combine the crackers with the butter until the crackers are moistened. Push the crust mixture onto the bottom of the pan. Use a layer of plastic and cover the pan. Chill while you prepare the filling.
2. Use a blender/food processor to combine ¼ cup of sugar, cream cheese, ¼ cup of milk, orange peel, and vanilla. Place a lid on the blender and mix until it's creamy smooth. Transfer the mixture into a holding container and put it to the side for now.
3. Next, combine the pumpkin with the remaining ¼ cup milk, the fat-free cream cheese, the rest of the ¼ cup sugar, and the pumpkin pie spice. Securely close the lid and blend until smooth.
4. Sprinkle the gelatin into the orange juice into a pan and let it marinate for five minutes. Simmer and stir using the low-temperature setting until the gelatin is liquified.
5. Combine one tablespoon of the gelatin mixture into the white cream cheese mixture and the remainder of the gelatin mixture into the pumpkin mixture.
6. Empty the pumpkin mixture over the chilled crust. Slowly empty the white cream cheese mixture over the pumpkin mixture. Swirl the pumpkin and white blends.
7. Use a layer of foil to chill the cake overnight before serving.
8. Gently 'break' the cheesecake from the sides of the pan and pop it out. Slice it into wedges to serve.

Phyllo-Crusted Melon Cheesecake

Servings Provided: 10

Time Required: 4 hours 50 minutes

Macro Counts - Each Serving:

- ❖ Calories: 137
- ❖ Carbs: 15.8 g
- ❖ Sugar: 8.5 g
- ❖ Fiber: 1.1 g
- ❖ Chol: 14 mg
- ❖ Prot.: 4.3 g
- ❖ Sodium: 159.4 mg
- ❖ Fat Content: 6.2 g (Saturated: 4.2 g)
  D.E.:
- ❖ Fat: 1
- ❖ Other Carbohydrate: 1

Ingredients Needed:

- ❖ Frozen phyllo dough - thawed (8 sheets)
- ❖ Toasted wheat germ (3 tbsp.)
- ❖ Water (3 tbsp.)
- ❖ Unflavored gelatin (1.5 tsp.)
- ❖ Light cream cheese - softened (8 oz. pkg.)
- ❖ Light dairy sour cream (.5 cup)
- ❖ Powdered sugar (1 tbsp.)
- ❖ Frozen light whipped dessert topping (half of 8 oz. container)
- ❖ Assorted melon pieces (3 cups)
- ❖ Fresh raspberries (.25 cup)
- ❖ Fresh thyme and/or oregano (1 sprig)
- ❖ Butter-flavor nonstick cooking spray (as needed)
- ❖ Non-stick cooking oil spray (as needed)
- ❖ Suggested: 9-inch tart pan with a removable bottom (1 to 2 inches deep)

Preparation Technique:

1. Thaw the whipped topping.
2. Thinly slice the melon into wedges - removing the peel.
3. Coat the tart pan using a nonstick cooking spray.
4. Tip: While you are preparing each of the tarts, cover the rest of the sheets with a plastic wrap to keep them fresh.
5. Remove a sheet from the package of dough. Lightly spritz it with the cooking spray.
6. Add another sheet of the phyllo dough and also spray it.
7. Gently push the dough into the tart pan, extending it to the edge of the pan. Dust the crust with the wheat germ (1 tbsp.).
8. Lightly spray and layer another two sheets of the dough, placing it across the phyllo in the pan (criss-cross fashion). Sprinkle using another tablespoon of the wheat germ.
9. Add two more sheets of the phyllo dough, cooking spray, and wheat germ, placing the rectangles in the pan at an angle to completely cover the bottom of the pan.
10. Once more, add the last two sheets of dough and nonstick cooking spray. Turn under the edges of phyllo dough to form a border.Bake until the crust is lightly browned (10-12 min.). Cool in a pan on a wire rack.
11. Prepare the filling: Pour the water into the pan and add the gelatin (*don't stir*). Wait for five minutes until it softens.
12. Cook and stir using the low-temperature setting until the gelatin liquefies. Wait for it to slightly cool.
13. Use the medium-speed setting of an electric mixer to beat the sour cream with the cream cheese and powdered sugar until smooth. Add in the gelatin mixture, pulsing until combined. Lastly, mix in the whipped topping.
14. Scoop the batter into the cooled crust. Cover and chill for four hours to one day.
15. When you're ready to enjoy it, arrange the wedges of raspberries and melon balls over the cheesecake.
16. Garnish as desired with fresh oregano and thyme. Slice into wedges to serve.

Protein Cheesecake

Servings Provided: 2

Time Required: 1 hour

Macro Counts - Each Serving:

- ❖ Calories: 165
- ❖ Carbs: 6 g
- ❖ Sugar: 3.5 g
- ❖ Chol: 12 mg
- ❖ Prot.: 32.5 g
- ❖ Sodium: 560 mg
- ❖ Fat Content: 0.5 g (Saturated: -0- g)
- ❖ Net Carbs: 6 g

Ingredients Needed:

- ❖ Low fat cottage cheese (8.5 oz.)
- ❖ Egg whites (2)
- ❖ Vanilla protein powder (1 scoop)
- ❖ Stevia (1 tbsp.)
- ❖ Vanilla extract (1 tsp.)
- ❖ S.F. Strawberry Jell-O (1 serving)
- ❖ Water

Preparation Technique:

- ❖ Warm the oven to 325° F/163° C.
- ❖ Prepare the Jell-O per the package directions and pop it in the freezer.
- ❖ Blend the cottage cheese with the egg whites until the consistency is smooth.
- ❖ Empty the blended mixture into a mixing container and whisk it with the protein powder, vanilla extract, and stevia.
- ❖ Scoop the batter into a small nonstick pan and bake for 25 minutes.
- ❖ Extinguish the heat in the oven, leaving the cake in it while it cools down. Once the oven has cooled, remove the cheesecake.

❖ When the Jell-O is almost set, pour it over the cheesecake.

❖ Let the cake become firm in the fridge for about 10-12 hours before serving.

Raspberry & Chocolate Cheesecake

Servings Provided: 12

Time Required: 25 minutes + chill time

Macro Counts - Each Serving:

- ❖ Calories: 237
- ❖ Carbs: 27 g
- ❖ Sugar: 17 g
- ❖ Fiber: 2 g
- ❖ Chol: 14 mg
- ❖ Prot.: 14 g
- ❖ Sodium: 576 mg
- ❖ Fat Content: 7 g (Saturated: 4 g)
  D.E:
- ❖ Starch: 2
- ❖ Fat: 1
- ❖ Lean Meat: 1

Ingredients Needed:

- ❖ Graham cracker crumbs (.75 cup)
- ❖ Unflavored gelatin (1 envelope)
- ❖ Water (1 cup - *cold*)
- ❖ Melted butter (2 tbsp.)
- ❖ Semisweet chocolate (4 oz.)
- ❖ F.F. cream cheese (4 pkg. @ 8 oz. each)
- ❖ Sugar (.5 cup)
- ❖ Sugar substitute (equal to 1 cup sugar)
- ❖ Baking cocoa (.25 cup)
- ❖ Vanilla extract (2 tsp.)
- ❖ Fresh raspberries (2 cups)

Preparation Technique:

1. Crush the cracker crumbs and mix with the butter, pressing it into the base of a greased nine-inch springform pan.
2. Set a timer to bake at 375° Fahrenheit or 191° Celsius until nicely browned (8-10 min.). Wait for a few minutes for it to cool in the pan over a wire rack.
3. Coarsely chop the chocolate. Prepare the filling in a saucepan.
4. Pour the gelatin into chilled water and wait for one minute. Warm it using the low-temperature setting, stirring until gelatin is thoroughly liquified. Mix in the semisweet chocolate, stirring until melted.
5. In another container, combine the sugar substitute with the cream cheese and sugar until smooth. Slowly, mix the chocolate mixture with the cocoa, beating in the vanilla. Empty the mixture into the crust. Pop it in the fridge until firm (2-3 hrs.).
6. Arrange raspberries on top of the cheesecake. Loosen the edges of the cake from the pan using a knife. Serve as desired.

Chapter 8

Tasty Fruits & Tarts

Fruity Desserts

Apple Crumble With Oats - Vegetarian

Servings Provided: 6

Time Required: 1 hour

Macro Counts - Each Serving:

- ❖ Calories: 148
- ❖ Carbs: 29.7 g
- ❖ Sugar: 16.5 g
- ❖ Fiber: 3.9 g
- ❖ Chol: 5.1 mg
- ❖ Protein: 2.7 g
- ❖ Sodium: 20.2 mg
- ❖ Fat Content: 3 g (Saturated: 1 g)
  D.E.:
- ❖ Starch: ½
- ❖ Fat: ½
- ❖ Fruit: 1
- ❖ Other Carbohydrate: ½

Ingredients Needed:

- ❖ Regular rolled oats (.5 cup)

❖ Whole-wheat pastry flour (2 tbsp.)

❖ Brown sugar - divided & packed (2 tbsp. + 1 tbsp.)

❖ Ground cinnamon (.5 tsp.)

❖ Cold butter (1 tbsp.)

❖ Golden Delicious apples (3 medium)

❖ Fresh lemon juice (1 tbsp.)

❖ Water (2 tbsp.)

❖ Frozen or low-fat vanilla yogurt (8 oz. container)

Preparation Technique:

1. Warm the oven to reach 350° Fahrenheit or 177 ° Celsius.
2. Combine the oats with the flour, cinnamon, and two tablespoons of brown sugar. Thoroughly stir until combined.
3. Cube and add the butter. Work it in until the mixture begins to form clumps.
4. Core the apples and slice them into thin wedges.
5. Toss the apples with the lemon juice, water, and remaining one tablespoon of brown sugar in a big mixing container. Scoop the apple mixture to a nine-inch pie plate. Sprinkle the oat mixture evenly over the apples.
6. Bake until the topping is nicely browned and the apples are juicy tender (40-45 min.). Serve warm with yogurt if desired.

Chili-Lime Grilled Pineapple

Servings Provided: 6

Time Required: 15 minutes

Macro Counts - Each Serving:

- ❖ Calories: 97
- ❖ Carbs: 20 g
- ❖ Sugar: 17 g
- ❖ Fiber: 1 g
- ❖ Chol: -0- mg
- ❖ Prot.: 1 g
- ❖ Sodium: 35 mg
- ❖ Fat Content: 2 g (Saturated: -0- g)
  D.E:
- ❖ Starch: ½
- ❖ Fat: ½
- ❖ Fruit: ½

Ingredients Needed:

- ❖ Fresh pineapple (1)
- ❖ Brown sugar (3 tbsp.)
- ❖ Lime juice (1 tbsp.)
- ❖ Honey/agave nectar (1 tbsp.)
- ❖ Olive oil (1 tbsp.)
- ❖ Chili powder (1.5 tsp.)
- ❖ Salt (1 dash)

Preparation Technique:

1. Peel the pineapple, removing any eyes from the fruit. Cut lengthwise into six wedges; remove the core. Mix the rest of the fixings until blended in a mixing container.
2. Brush the pineapple with half of the glaze; reserve the remaining mixture for basting.

3. Cover and grill the pineapple using the medium-temperature setting. Or - broil about four inches from the burner's heat for two to four minutes per side or until lightly browned, occasionally basting with the reserved glaze.

Cranberry Slow-Cooked Stuffed Apples

Servings Provided: 5

Time Required: 4 hours 10 minutes

Macro Counts - Each Serving:

- ❖ Calories: 136
- ❖ Carbs: 31 g
- ❖ Sugar: 25 g
- ❖ Fiber: 4 g
- ❖ Sodium: 6 mg
- ❖ Chol: -0- mg
- ❖ Fat Content: 2 g (Saturated: -0- g)
- ❖ Protein: 1 g
  D.E:
- ❖ Starch: 1
- ❖ Fruit: 1

Ingredients Needed:

- ❖ Apples (5 medium)
- ❖ Fresh or frozen cranberries (.33 cup)
- ❖ Chopped walnuts (2 tbsp.)
- ❖ Ground nutmeg (.125 tsp.)
- ❖ Packed brown sugar (.25 cup)
- ❖ Ground cinnamon (.25 tsp.)
- ❖ Optional: Vanilla ice cream or Whipped cream
- ❖ Also Needed: 5-quart slow cooker

Preparation Technique:

1. Thaw and chop the berries.
2. Core the apples, leaving bottoms intact. Peel the top 1/3 of each apple and put it into the cooker.

3. Mix the brown sugar with cinnamon, nutmeg, walnuts, and cranberries. Scoop it over the apples.
4. Securely close the lid and set the setting on low until apples are tender (4-5 hrs.).
5. Garnish and serve as desired.

Fruity Pizza

Servings Provided: 16

Time Required: 35 minutes + cooling time

Macro Counts - Each Serving:

- ❖ Calories: 170
- ❖ Carbs: 20 g
- ❖ Fiber: 1 g
- ❖ Sugar: 13 g
- ❖ Sodium: 120 mg
- ❖ Prot.: 3 g
- ❖ Chol: 25 mg
- ❖ Fat Content: 9 g (Saturated: 6 g)
  D.E:
- ❖ Starch: 1
- ❖ Fat: 1 ½
- ❖ Fruit: ½

Ingredients Needed:

- ❖ Confectioners' sugar (.25 cup)
- ❖ A.P. flour (1 cup)
- ❖ Cubed cold butter (.5 cup)
- ❖ *The Glaze*:
- ❖ Lemon juice (1 tsp.)
- ❖ Cornstarch (5 tsp.)
- ❖ Pineapple juice - unsweetened (1.25 cup)
  The Toppings:
- ❖ Reduced-fat cream cheese (8 oz. pkg.)
- ❖ Sugar (.33 cup)
- ❖ Vanilla extract (1 tsp.)
- ❖ Fresh strawberries (2 cups - halved)
- ❖ Mandarin oranges - drained (11 oz. can)

* Fresh blueberries (1 cup)
* Also Needed: 12-inch pizza pan

Preparation Technique:

1. Warm the oven to 350° Fahrenheit or 177 ° Celsius.
2. Whisk or sift the flour with the confectioners' sugar. Cut/mix in the butter until the mixture is crumbly. Work and press the mixture into an ungreased pan.
3. Bake it until very lightly browned (9-12 min.). Cool it thoroughly on a wire rack.
4. Use a small saucepan to mix glaze fixings until smooth. Wait for it to boil. Simmer and stir until thickened (about 2 min.). Cool slightly.
5. In another container, cream the sugar with the cream cheese and vanilla until it's creamy. Spread it over the crust and top with berries and oranges. Drizzle with the glaze and refrigerate until cold.

High-Protein Berry Crumble

Servings Provided: 1

Time Required: 20 minutes

Macro Counts - Each Serving:

- ❖ Calories: 320
- ❖ Carbs: 34.8 g
- ❖ Sugar: 7.7 g
- ❖ Fiber: 11.6 g
- ❖ Chol: 12.5 mg
- ❖ Protein: 29.6 g
- ❖ Sodium: 71.7 mg
- ❖ Fat Content: 8.6 g (Saturated: g)
- ❖ Net Carbs: 23.2

Ingredients Needed:

- ❖ Fresh or frozen raspberries/mixed berries (1 cup/125 g)
- ❖ Stevia (1 tsp.)
- ❖ Vanilla protein powder (1 scoop)
- ❖ Oats (.25 cup/20g)
- ❖ Lemon juice (2 tbsp.)
- ❖ Almonds (10)
- ❖ Also Needed: Small Pyrex oven dish

Preparation Technique:

1. Set the oven temperature at 350° F/177 ° C.
2. Toss the berries into the oven dish and dust with the Stevia over the top.
3. Combine the protein powder with oats and lemon juice. Chop the almonds into small pieces and mix them with the crumble.
4. Spread the crumble over the berries.
5. Set a timer to bake for 15 minutes. Adjust the temperature setting to broil and bake the crumble for another one to two minutes until the top is browned to your liking.
6. Place the pan on the countertop to cool slightly before serving.

Mango Tiramisù - Made Your Way

Servings Provided: 8

Time Required: 8 ½ hours

Macro Counts - Each Serving:

- ❖ 2/3 cup portion:
- ❖ Calories: 147
- ❖ Carbs: 27 g
- ❖ Fiber: 1 g
- ❖ Sugar: 14 g
- ❖ Chol: 37 mg
- ❖ Prot.: 5 g
- ❖ Sodium: 35 mg
- ❖ Fat Content: 3 g (Saturated: 2 g)
  D.E.:
- ❖ Starch: 1
- ❖ Fat: ½
- ❖ Fruit: ½
- ❖ Other Carbohydrate: ½

Ingredients Needed:

- ❖ Mangoes - frozen or refrigerated (16 oz.) or (2 medium + more for garnish)
- ❖ Light agave syrup (2 tbsp.)
- ❖ Almond extract (.25 tsp.)
- ❖ Frozen light whipped topping - thawed (1 cup)
- ❖ N.F. Greek yogurt - vanilla (1 cup)
- ❖ Crisp ladyfingers- Ex. Alessi Biscotti Savoiardi - broken into 1-inch pieces (12)

Preparation Technique:

1. Cube and add half of the mango in a food processor and pulse until it's creamy. Empty the puree into a small bowl. Mix in agave syrup and almond extract.
2. Pulse the remaining mango in the food processor until coarsely chopped. Set aside.

3. Gently fold whipped topping into yogurt in another small bowl. Sprinkle half the ladyfinger pieces into a two-quart shallow baking dish. Spoon half the mango puree and half the yogurt mixture over them. Top with the chopped mango.
4. Layer on the remaining ladyfingers, puree, and yogurt.
5. Gently fold whipped topping into yogurt in another small bowl. Sprinkle half the ladyfinger pieces into the baking dish. Spoon half the mango puree and half the yogurt mixture over them. Top with the chopped mango.
6. Layer on the remaining ladyfingers, puree, and yogurt.

Marinated Oranges

Servings Provided: 4

Time Required: 15 minutes + marinate time

Macro Counts - Each Serving:

- ❖ ¾ cup portions:
- ❖ Calories: 86
- ❖ Carbs: 20 g
- ❖ Sugar: 16 g
- ❖ Fiber: -0- g
- ❖ Chol: -0- mg
- ❖ Prot.: 1 g
- ❖ Sodium: 7 mg
- ❖ Fat Content: -0- g
  D.E:
- ❖ Fruit: 1 ½

Ingredients Needed:

- ❖ Grated orange zest (1 tbsp.)
- ❖ Vanilla extract (1 tsp.)
- ❖ Zested lemon (1 tsp.)
- ❖ Orange juice (1 cup)
- ❖ Sugar (1 tbsp.)
- ❖ Lemon juice (1 tbsp.)
  ****
- ❖ Medium oranges (4/about 3 cups)
- ❖ Optional: Lime zest strips & vanilla yogurt

Preparation Technique:

1. Mix the fixings up to the line (***), stirring until sugar is dissolved.
2. Peel and thinly slice the oranges. Add them to a glass bowl, and add the juice mixture.

3. Refrigerate, covered, until flavors are blended (2-3 hrs.). If desired, top with lime zest strips and serve with yogurt.

Picnic Berry Shortcakes

Servings Provided: 4

Time Required: 20 minutes + chill time

Macro Counts - Each Serving:

- ❖ Calories: 124
- ❖ Carbs: 29 g
- ❖ Sugar: 21 g
- ❖ Fiber: 3 g
- ❖ Chol: 10 mg
- ❖ Prot.: 2 g
- ❖ Sodium: 67 mg
- ❖ Fat Content: 1 g (Saturated: -0- g)
  D.E.:
- ❖ Starch: 1
- ❖ Fruit: 1

Ingredients Needed:

- ❖ Water (2 tbsp.)
- ❖ Sugar (2 tbsp.)
- ❖ Cornstarch (.5 tsp.)
- ❖ Fresh strawberries - divided (2 cups)
- ❖ Grated lime zest (.5 tsp.)
- ❖ Fresh blueberries (2 cups)
- ❖ Round sponge cakes (2 @ individually-sized)
- ❖ Optional: Whipped topping
- ❖ Also Needed: Wide-mouth half-pint canning jars (4)

Preparation Technique:

1. Use a saucepan to combine the cornstarch with the sugar. Pour in the water. Slice and add one cup of the strawberries and mash the mixture. Wait for it to boil and cook - stirring

until thickened (1-2 min.). Transfer the pan to a cool spot and mix in lime zest. Pour it into a small container and pop it into the fridge, covered until chilled.

2. Slice the sponge cakes crosswise into halves. Trim them to fit in the bottoms of the jars.

3. Toss the blueberries and the rest of the strawberries over the cakes. Pour the sauce over the tops and garnish to your liking.

Strawberry Nutella S'mores

Servings Provided: 1

Time Required: 10 minutes

Macro Counts - Each Serving:

- ❖ Calories: 76
- ❖ Carbs: 12.7 g
- ❖ Sugar: 7.7 g
- ❖ Fiber: 0.7 g
- ❖ Chol: 2 mg
- ❖ Protein: 0.8 g
- ❖ Sodium: 21.1 mg
- ❖ Fat Content: 2.6 g (Saturated: 0.8 g)
  D.E.:
- ❖ Starch: ½
- ❖ Other Carbohydrate: ½

Ingredients Needed:

- ❖ Marshmallow (1)
- ❖ Chocolate-hazelnut spread (.5 tsp.)
- ❖ Ladyfingers (2)
- ❖ Lemon thins (2)
- ❖ Strawberry slices (2)

Preparation Technique:

1. Toast the marshmallow over a fire.
2. Spread the chocolate-hazelnut spread over a lemon thin.
3. Top it off using the marshmallow, strawberry, and the second lemon thin.

Warm Spiced Apples

Servings Provided: 6

Time Required: 20 minutes

Macro Counts - Each Serving:

- 2/3 cup portions:
- Calories: 101
- Carbs: 26.9 g
- Sugar: 21.5 g
- Fiber: 3.8 g
- Chol: -0- mg
- Prot.: 0.4 g
- Sodium: 2.1 mg
- Fat Content: 0.3 g (Saturated: 0.1 g)
  D.E.:
- Other Carbohydrate: 1
- Fruit: 1

Ingredients Needed:

- Red-skinned cooking apples - ex. Jonathon or Rome (5 medium/about 7 cups)
- Water (.25 cup)
- Cinnamon (.5 tsp.)
- Ground nutmeg(.125 tsp./as desired)
- Honey (2 tbsp.)

Preparation Technique:

1. Remove the core, quarter, and thinly slice the apples.
2. Combine the apple slices with the water in a large skillet. Sprinkle with nutmeg and cinnamon. Once boiling, lower the temperature setting.
3. Place a lid on the pot and simmer until the apples are just tender, stirring once or twice (3 min.).
4. Drizzle with honey and toss to coat.
5. Scoop the serve warm in six individual serving bowls.

Tarts

Ginger Plum Tart

Servings Provided: 8

Time Required: 35 minutes

Macro Counts - Each Serving:

- Calories: 190
- Carbs: 30 g
- Sugar: 14 g
- Fiber: 1 g
- Sodium: 198 mg
- Prot.: 2 g
- Chol: 5 mg
- Fat Content: 7 g (Saturated: 3 g)
  D.E.:
- Starch: 1 ½
- Fat: 1
- Fruit: ½

Ingredients Needed:

- Refrigerated pie crust (12-inch sheet)
- Cornstarch (1 tbsp.)
- Sugar (3 tbsp.)
- Crystallized ginger (2 tsp.)
- Egg white (1 large)
- Water (1 tbsp.)

Preparation Technique:

1. Slice the plums and finely chop the ginger. Cover a baking tray using a sheet of parchment baking paper.
2. Set the oven to 400° Fahrenheit/204° Celsius.
3. Unroll the crust and place it on the prepared tray.

4. Toss the plums with cornstarch and sugar. Place them over the crust to within two inches of its edges and sprinkle with ginger. Fold the crust edge over plums, pleating as you go.
5. Whisk the egg white and water, making an egg wash to brush over the folded crust. Sprinkle with the rest of the sugar.
6. Bake until the crust is nicely browned (18-25 min.). Wait for it to cool in the pan.
7. Once it's cooled, serve as desired.

Pear Tart

Servings Provided: 12

Time Required: 40 minutes

Macro Counts - Each Serving:

- ❖ Calories: 199
- ❖ Carbs: 25 g
- ❖ Sugar: 18 g
- ❖ Fiber: 1 g
- ❖ Chol: 36 mg
- ❖ Protein: 4 g
- ❖ Fat Content: 9 g (Saturated: 5 g)
- ❖ Sodium: 112 mg
    D.E.:
- ❖ Starch: 1 ½
- ❖ Fat: 2

Ingredients Needed:

- ❖ Unchilled butter (3 tbsp.)
- ❖ Sugar (.5 cup)
- ❖ A.P. flour (.75 cup)
- ❖ Ground cinnamon (.75 tsp.)
- ❖ Finely chopped walnuts (.33 cup)
    The Filling:
- ❖ Reduced-fat cream cheese (8 oz. pkg.)
- ❖ Sugar - divided (.25 cup + 1 tbsp.)
- ❖ Unchille egg (1 large)
- ❖ Vanilla extract (1 tsp.)
- ❖ Reduced-sugar sliced pears (15 oz. can)
- ❖ Ground cinnamon (.25 tsp.)
- ❖ Also Needed: Nine-inch fluted tart pan & removable bottom.

Preparation Technique:

1. Set the oven to reach 425° F/218° C.
2. Thoroughly drain and thinly slice the pears. Mix the butter with the sugar and cinnamon until crumbly. Mix in the walnuts and flour. Work, pushing the dough mix into bottom and up sides of the pan coated with cooking spray.
3. Make the filling by mixing the cream cheese and sugar (¼ cup) until it's creamy.
4. Whisk in the egg and vanilla. Spread into the crust.
5. Arrange the sliced pears over the top. Mix the cinnamon and the rest of the sugar and sprinkle over the pears.
6. Bake for ten minutes. Adjust the oven's temperature setting to 350° Fahrenheit or 177 ° Celsius.
7. Bake until the filling is set (15 to 20 min.).
8. Cool it for one hour on a wire rack. Pop it into the fridge for a minimum of two hours before serving.

<h1 align="center">Chapter 9</h1>

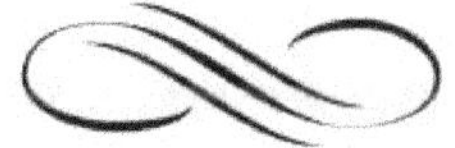

<h1 align="center">Brownies & Fudge</h1>

Applesauce Brownies

Servings Provided: 16

Time Required: 40 minutes

Macro Counts - Each Serving:

- ❖ Calories: 154
- ❖ Carbs: 22 g
- ❖ Sugar: 15 g
- ❖ Fiber: 1 g
- ❖ Chol: 21 mg
- ❖ Prot.: 2 g
- ❖ Sodium: 65 mg
- ❖ Fat Content: 7 g (Saturated: 3 g)
  D.E.:
- ❖ Starch: 1 ½
- ❖ Fat: 1 ½

Ingredients Needed:

- ❖ Unchilled butter - softened (.25 cup)
- ❖ Sugar (.75 cup)
- ❖ Egg (1 large)
- ❖ Baking soda (.5 tsp.)

- A.P. flour (1 cup)
- Baking cocoa (1 tbsp.)
- Ground cinnamon (.5 tsp.)
- Applesauce (1 cup)
- The Topping:
- Chocolate chips (.5 cup)
- Chopped walnuts/pecans (.5 cup)
- Sugar (1 tbsp.)
- Needed: Eight-inch square baking pan

Preparation Technique:

1. Combine the butter with the sugar in a big mixing container. Beat and mix in the egg.
2. Sift to combine the cocoa with the baking soda, flour, and cinnamon. Slowly add and mix into the creamed mixture. Fold in the applesauce.
3. Spritz the baking tray using a portion of cooking oil spray and add the mix.
4. Toss and sprinkle the topping fixings over the batter.
5. Bake at 350° Fahrenheit or 177 ° Celsius until done (25 min.). Cool the brownies over a wire rack before cutting them into 16 squares.

Cream Cheese Swirl Brownies

Servings Provided: 12

Time Required: 45 minutes

Macro Counts - Each Serving:

- ❖ Calories: 172
- ❖ Carbs: 23 g
- ❖ Sugar: 18 g
- ❖ Chol: 36 mg
- ❖ Prot.: 4 g
- ❖ Sodium: 145 mg
- ❖ Fat Content: 8 g (Saturated: 5 g)
  D.E.:
- ❖ Starch: 1 ½
- ❖ Fat: 1 ½ fat

Ingredients Needed:

- ❖ Eggs - divided (3 large)
- ❖ Unchilled reduced-fat butter (6 tbsp.)
- ❖ Sugar - divided (1 cup)
- ❖ Baking cocoa (.25 cup)
- ❖ Vanilla extract (3 tsp.)
- ❖ A.P. flour (.5 cup)
- ❖ Reduced-fat cream cheese (8 oz. pkg.)
- ❖ Needed: 9-inch square baking pan

Preparation Technique:

1. Warm the oven to reach 350° F/177 ° C.
2. Separate two eggs (tossing the yolks), putting each white in a separate bowl, and place it to the side for now.
3. Combine and mix 3/4 cup sugar with the butter until crumbly. Whisk and mix in one egg white, the remaining whole egg, and vanilla - mixing until it's thoroughly combined.

4. Whisk or sift the flour and cocoa, slowly adding it to the egg mixture until blended. Empty it into the baking pan coated with cooking spray; set aside.

5. Mix the cream cheese with the rest of the sugar until smooth. Fold in the second egg white. Drop by rounded tablespoonfuls over the batter, cutting through the batter with a knife to swirl.

6. Bake until set and edges pull away from the pan's sides (25-30 min.). Cool on a wire rack and serve.

Easy No-Bake Chocolate Fudge - Keto- Vegan-Friendly

Servings Provided: 40 squares

Time Required: 5 minutes + chill time 2 hours

Macro Counts - Each Serving:

- ❖ Calories: 122
- ❖ Carbs: 5.85 g
- ❖ Sugar: 2.97 g
- ❖ Fiber: 2.28g
- ❖ Prot.: 1.325 g
- ❖ Sodium: mg
- ❖ Fat Content: 11 g (Saturated: 8.8 g)

Ingredients Needed:

- ❖ Coconut butter (1.5 cups)
- ❖ Full-fat coconut milk (13.66 fl. oz. can)
- ❖ Bittersweet chocolate chips (10 oz.)
- ❖ Optional Topping: Flaked/coarse sea salt
- ❖ Also Suggested: 8 by 8-inch baking pan

Preparation Technique:

1. Line the baking pan with a layer of foil or waxed paper.
2. Melt the coconut butter in a saucepan using the low-temperature setting.
3. Mix in the chips and milk. Let the mixture simmer, frequently stirring until the chocolate has melted.
4. Empty the batter into the prepared baking pan. Drizzle with sea salt and pop it into the fridge until it's set (2 hrs.). Slice and serve.

Super-Spud Brownies

Servings Provided: 16

Time Required: 40 minutes

Macro Counts - Each Serving:

- ❖ Calories: 150
- ❖ Carbs: 19 g
- ❖ Sugar: 13 g
- ❖ Chol: 27 mg
- ❖ Prot.: 2 g
- ❖ Sodium: 68 mg
- ❖ Fat Content: 8 g (Saturated: 1 g)
  D.E.:
- ❖ Starch: 1
- ❖ Fat: 1 ½

Ingredients Needed:

- ❖ Mashed potatoes (.75 cup)
- ❖ Sugar (.5 cup)
- ❖ Brown sugar - tightly packed (.5 cup)
- ❖ Eggs (2 large)
- ❖ Canola oil (.5 cup)
- ❖ Vanilla extract (1 tsp.)
- ❖ A.P. flour (.5 cup)
- ❖ Salt (.125 tsp.)
- ❖ Cocoa powder (.33 cup)
- ❖ Baking powder (.5 tsp.)
- ❖ Optional: Chopped pecans (.5 cup)
- ❖ Confectioners' sugar
- ❖ Suggested: 9-inch square baking tray

Preparation Technique:

1. Combine the mashed potatoes with the sugars, eggs, oil, and vanilla.
2. Sift the flour with the salt, cocoa, and baking powder; slowly adding the mixture into the potato mixture. Fold in the pecans and pour into a greased pan.
3. Bake at 350° Fahrenheit or 177 ° Celsius until a toothpick inserted in the center comes out clean (for 23-27 min.). Put the pan on a wire rack to cool.
4. Sprinkle using confectioners' sugar. Cut into 16 bars. Serve as desired.

Chapter 10

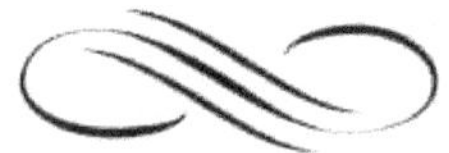

Cookie Favorites

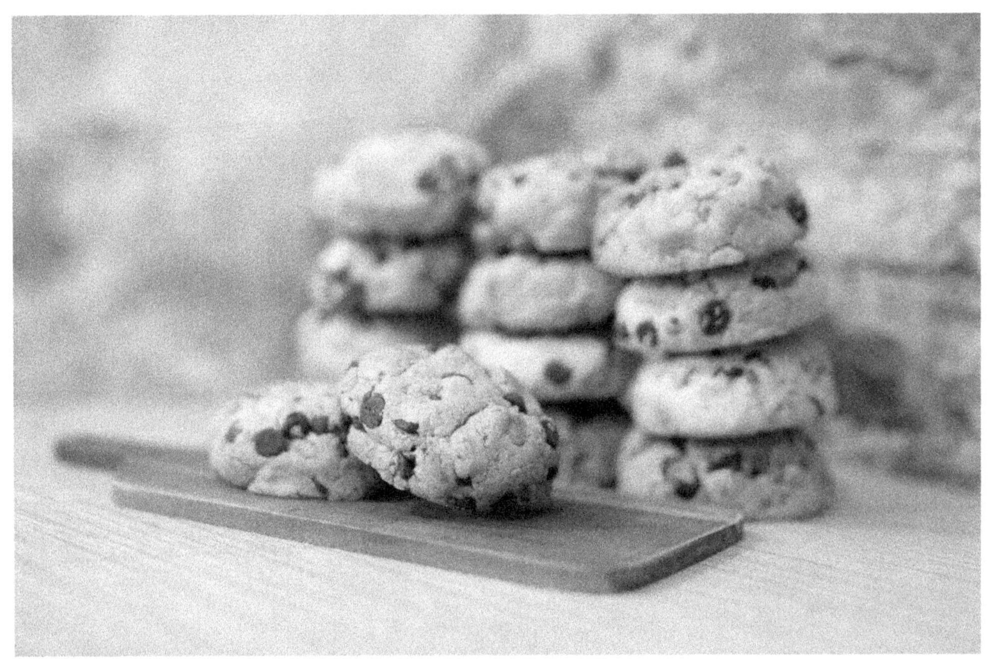

Servings Provided: 3 d0zen

Time Required: 35 minutes

Macro Counts - Each Serving:

- ❖ Calories: 69
- ❖ Carbs: 10 g
- ❖ Sugar: 6 g
- ❖ Fiber: -0- g
- ❖ Sodium: 50 mg
- ❖ Protein: 1 g

- ❖ Chol: 10 mg
- ❖ Fat Content: 3 g (Saturated: 2 g)
  D.E.:
- ❖ Starch: ½
- ❖ Fat: ½

Ingredients Needed:

- ❖ Unchilled butter (.33 cup)
- ❖ Sugar (.5 cup)
- ❖ Unchilled egg (1 large)
- ❖ Vanilla extract (.5 tsp.)
- ❖ Mashed ripe banana (.5 cup)
- ❖ A.P. flour (1.25 cups)
- ❖ Bak. powder (1 tsp.)
- ❖ Salt (.25 tsp.)
- ❖ Bak. soda (.125 tsp.)
- ❖ Semisweet chocolate chips (1 cup)

Preparation Technique:

- ❖ Mix the sugar with the butter until fluffy. Whisk and add in the egg, banana, and vanilla. Sift or whisk the flour with the baking powder, salt, and baking soda, slowly adding it into the creamed mixture. Fold in the chocolate chips.
- ❖ Drop by tablespoonfuls about two inches apart onto baking trays coated with cooking oil spray.
- ❖ Bake at 350° Fahrenheit/177 ° Celsius until the edges are browned (13-16 min.). Transfer the pans to wire racks to cool.
- ❖ Serve and enjoy them anytime.

Carrot Cookie Bites

Servings Provided: 7 dozen

Time Required: 25 minutes

Macro Counts - Each Serving:

- ❖ Calories: 50
- ❖ Carbs: 6 g
- ❖ Sugar: 3 g
- ❖ Protein: 1 g
- ❖ Chol: 5 mg
- ❖ Sodium: 24 mg
- ❖ Fat Content: 2 g (Saturated: -0- g)
  D.E.:
- ❖ Starch: ½
- ❖ Fat: ½

Ingredients Needed:

- ❖ Shortening (.66 cup)
- ❖ Brown sugar - tightly packed (1 cup)
- ❖ Unchilled large eggs (2)
- ❖ Buttermilk (.5 cup)
- ❖ Vanilla extract (1 tsp.)
- ❖ A.P. flour (2 cups)
- ❖ Salt (.5 tsp.)
- ❖ Bak. soda (.25 tsp.)
- ❖ Ground cloves (.25 tsp.)
- ❖ Bak. powder (.25 tsp.)
- ❖ Ground nutmeg (.25 tsp.)
- ❖ Cinnamon (1 tsp.)
- ❖ Shredded carrots (1 cup)
- ❖ Oats - Quick-cooking type (2 cups)
- ❖ Pecans (.5 cup)

Preparation Technique:

1. Combine the shortening with the brown sugar until light and fluffy (5-7 min.). Whisk and mix in the eggs with the buttermilk and vanilla. Whisk the flour with the salt, baking powder, cinnamon, cloves, baking soda, and nutmeg. Slowly mix it into the creamed mixture.
2. Chop and mix in the pecans, carrots, and oats.
3. Scoop and drop the dough by rounded teaspoonfuls onto ungreased baking sheets (2 in. apart).
4. Set the timer to bake at 375° Fahrenheit or 191° Celsius until lightly browned (6-8 min.). Place the pans onto wire racks to cool.
5. You have a freezer option. Scoop them by teaspoonfuls onto parchment-lined baking sheets. Freeze until firm. Transfer the cookie dough balls to zipper-type bags or other freezer containers; seal tightly and freeze for up to three months. To bake, place the frozen dough two inches apart on ungreased baking sheets.
6. Bake at 375° Fahrenheit or 191° Celsius until browned for 10-15 minutes (since the dough is chilled). Transfer them onto wire racks to cool.

Carrot Raisin Cookies

Servings Provided: 36

Time Required: 50 minutes

Macro Counts - Each Serving:

- ❖ Calories: 98
- ❖ Carbs: 14 g
- ❖ Fiber: 1 g
- ❖ Sugar: 8 g
- ❖ Chol: 12 mg
- ❖ Prot.: 2 g
- ❖ Fat Content: 4 g (Saturated: 2 g)
- ❖ Sodium: 115 mg
  D.E.:
- ❖ Starch: ½
- ❖ Fat: 1/2
- ❖ Other Carbohydrate: ½

Ingredients Needed:

- ❖ Unchilled butter (.5 cup)
- ❖ Brown sugar (1 cup - packed)
- ❖ Ground cinnamon (1 tsp.)
- ❖ Salt (.25 tsp.)
- ❖ Bak. soda (2 tsp.)
- ❖ Ground ginger (1 tsp.)
- ❖ Egg (1)
- ❖ Unsweetened applesauce (.25 cup)
- ❖ Vanilla (1 tsp.)
- ❖ Whole wheat flour (2 cups)
- ❖ Carrots, finely shredded (1 cup/2 medium)
- ❖ Raisins (.75 cup)
- ❖ Finely chopped walnuts (.75 cup)

Preparation Technique:

1. Warm the oven to reach 375° F/191° C.
2. Combine the butter using an electric mixer using the medium speed setting for ½ minute.
3. Measure and mix in the baking soda, brown sugar, cinnamon, ginger, and salt, thoroughly mixing until combined.
4. Mix in the egg, applesauce, and vanilla. Fold in any remaining flour, raisins, carrots, and walnuts - just until combined.
5. Drop by slightly rounded teaspoons two inches apart onto ungreased baking trays.
6. Bake until the edges are firm (8-9 min.).
7. Place the cookies onto a wire rack to thoroughly cool.

Chocolate Chip Cookies

Servings Provided: 40

Time Required: 45 minutes

Macro Counts - Each Serving:

- ❖ Calories: 78
- ❖ Fiber: 1 g
- ❖ Carbs: 10 g
- ❖ Chol: 3 mg
- ❖ Prot.: 2 g
- ❖ Sodium: 47 mg
- ❖ Fat Content: 4 g (Saturated: 2 g)
  D.E.:
- ❖ Fat: ½
- ❖ Carb Choices: ½
- ❖ Other Carb: ½

Ingredients Needed:

- ❖ Boiling water (.5 cup)
- ❖ Raisins (1 cup)
- ❖ Peanut butter (.5 cup)
- ❖ Unchilled butter (.25 cup)
- ❖ Sugar (.5 cup)
- ❖ Baking soda (.5 tsp.)
- ❖ Refrigerated or frozen egg product - thawed (.5 cup)
- ❖ Ground cinnamon (1 tsp.)
- ❖ Vanilla (1 tsp.)
- ❖ A.P. flour (.5 cup)
- ❖ Regular rolled oats (1.25 cups)
- ❖ Chocolate chunks - semi-sweet (1 cup)

Preparation Technique:

1. Warm the oven temperature to reach 350° Fahrenheit/177 ° Celsius.
2. Cover cookie sheets with parchment baking paper, if desired.
3. Toss the raisins and boiling water in a mixing dish and set it aside.
4. Cream the peanut butter with the butter or beat with an electric mixer using the medium-speed setting for ½ minute.
5. Add the cinnamon, sugar substitute, baking soda, egg product, and vanilla. Blend until incorporated.
6. Mix in the flour, and lastly, the oats.
7. Drain the raisins and combine with the chocolate pieces, adding them into the oat mixture.
8. Drop the batter by rounded teaspoons onto the prepared baking trays.
9. Bake them until lightly browned (10 min.).
10. Place the pans onto wire racks to cool.

Keto Vegan Pumpkin Cookies

Servings Provided: 12

Time Required: 40 minutes

Macro Counts - Each Serving:

- ❖ Calories: 156
- ❖ Carbs: 5.4 g
- ❖ Fiber: 2.3 g
- ❖ Sugar: 1.1 g
- ❖ Chol: -0- mg
- ❖ Prot.: 4.2 g
- ❖ Sodium: 94.1 mg
- ❖ Fat Content: 14.1 g (Saturated: 4.4 g)
- ❖ Net Carbs: 3.1 g

Ingredients Needed:

- ❖ Almond flour (2 cups)
- ❖ Bak. powder (.5 tsp.)
- ❖ Sea salt (.5 tsp.)
- ❖ Flaxseed powder (1 tbsp.)
- ❖ Water (3 tbsp.)
- ❖ Unsweetened pumpkin puree (.5 cup)
- ❖ Coconut oil (.25 cup)
- ❖ Coconut oil (1 tsp./as needed)
- ❖ Vanilla extract (1 tsp.)
- ❖ Brown erythritol (.5 cup)
- ❖ Ground cinnamon (2 tsp.)
- ❖ To Garnish: Brown erythritol (4 tsp.)

Preparation Technique:

1. Warm the oven at 350° Fahrenheit/177 ° Celsius.
2. Prepare a cookie tray with a layer of parchment baking paper.

3. Sift the almond flour with the salt and baking powder in a mixing container.

4. Prepare a "flax egg" by mixing one tablespoon of flax powder and three tablespoons of water in a mixing cup or another container. Wait for five minutes. (Use one egg if not vegan.)

5. Add the flax egg with the pumpkin puree, melted coconut oil, and vanilla extract into a mixing container, whisking until smooth.

6. Add the erythritol to the wet fixings. Stir until well-combined, and most of the sweetener granules are liquified.

7. Combine the wet fixings to the almond flour mixture until the dough sticks together. (Add small amounts of almond flour if it's too sticky).

8. Oil your hands and roll out the dough (2 tbsp. at a time) into 12 balls and place on the baking sheet. Use a fork to press each ball down crosswise until they're about ½-inch thick.

9. Bake until they're just starting to brown and turn golden (15-20 min.).

10. Transfer the tray to the countertop and sprinkle with cinnamon and brown erythritol while warm.

11. Cool them on the cookie tray for 20 minutes. Gently move them onto a wire cooling rack to finish cooling to serve.

Molasses-Crackle Cookies

Servings Provided: 2.5 dozen

Time Required: 30 minutes + chill time

Macro Counts - Each Serving:

- ❖ Calories: 77
- ❖ Carbs: 14 g
- ❖ Sugar: 7 g
- ❖ Fiber: 1 g
- ❖ Chol: 7 mg
- ❖ Prot.: 1 g
- ❖ Sodium: 106 mg
- ❖ Fat Content: 2 g (Saturated: -0- g)
  D.E.:
- ❖ Starch: 1

Ingredients Needed:

- ❖ Canola oil (.25 cup)
- ❖ Egg (1 large)
- ❖ Sugar (.66 cup)
- ❖ Molasses (.33 cup)
- ❖ Ground cloves (.25 tsp.)
- ❖ White whole wheat flour (2 cups)
- ❖ Bak. soda (1.5 tsp.)
- ❖ Cinnamon (1 tsp.)
- ❖ Ground ginger (.25 tsp.)
- ❖ Salt (.5 tsp.)
- ❖ Confectioners' sugar (1 tbsp.)

Preparation Technique:

1. Mix the sugar with the oil until blended. Whisk and mix in the egg and molasses.

2. Whisk the flour with the salt, cloves, baking soda, ginger, and cinnamon. Mix it into the sugar mixture.

3. Cover the container and put it into the refrigerator to chill for a minimum of two hours.

4. Warm the oven temperature to reach 350° F/177 ° C.

5. Shape the dough into one-inch balls and roll them in confectioners' sugar.

6. Arrange them about two inches apart onto baking trays coated with cooking spray.

7. Fatten them slightly to bake for seven to nine minutes or until they're firm. Transfer the cookies to wire racks to cool. Serve as desired.

Oatmeal Cookies for the Holidays

Servings Provided: 6 dozen

Time Required: 45 minutes

Macro Counts - Each Serving:

- ❖ Calories: 56
- ❖ Carbs: 11 g
- ❖ Sugar: 6 g
- ❖ Fiber: 1 g
- ❖ Chol: 5 mg
- ❖ Prot.: 1 g
- ❖ Sodium: 40 mg
- ❖ Fat Content: 1 g (Saturated: 1 g)
  D.E.:
- ❖ Starch: 1

Ingredients Needed:

- ❖ Hot water (2 tbsp.)
- ❖ Ground flaxseed (1 tbsp.)
- ❖ Pitted dried plums (1 cup)
- ❖ Dates (1 cup)
- ❖ Raisins (.5 cup)
- ❖ Unchilled butter (.o.33 cup)
- ❖ Brown sugar (.75 cup - packed tight)
- ❖ Egg (1 large)
- ❖ Vanilla extract (2 tsp.)
- ❖ Unsweetened applesauce (.5 cup)
- ❖ Maple syrup (.25 cup)
- ❖ Grated orange zest (1 tbsp.)
- ❖ Oats - quick-cooking (3 cups)
- ❖ A.P. flour (1 cup)
- ❖ Baking soda (1 tsp.)

- ❖ Whole wheat flour (.5 cup)
- ❖ Ground nutmeg & cloves (.25 tsp. each)
- ❖ Salt (.5 tsp.)
- ❖ Cinnamon (1 tsp.)

Preparation Technique:

1. Combine water and flaxseed. Chop the dates and plums.
2. In another container, combine the plums, dates, and raisins. Pour in boiling water. Let the flaxseed and plum mixtures stand for ten minutes.
3. Meanwhile, combine the brown sugar with the butter until light and fluffy.
4. Mix in the whisked egg and vanilla. Beat in the applesauce, maple syrup, and orange zest. Combine the oats with both flours, salt, baking soda, cinnamon, nutmeg, and cloves. Slowly add to the creamed mixture. Drain the plum mixture; stir the plum and flaxseed into the dough.
5. Drop by rounded teaspoonfuls onto lightly greased baking trays (two inches apart). Bake at 350° Fahrenheit or 177 ° Celsius until set (8-11 min.).
6. Cool the cookies for about ten minutes. Remove them from the pans to wire racks.

Oatmeal & Peanut Butter Cookies

Servings Provided: 24

Time Required: 20 minutes

Macro Counts - Each Serving:

- ❖ Calories: 67
- ❖ Carbs: 8 g
- ❖ Fiber: 1 g
- ❖ Sugar: 5 g
- ❖ Chol: 9 mg
- ❖ Prot.: 2 g
- ❖ Sodium: 57 mg
- ❖ Fat Content: 3 g (Saturated: 1 g)
  D.E.:
- ❖ Starch: ½
- ❖ Fat: ½

Ingredients Needed:

- ❖ Peanut butter - chunky-style (.5 cup)
- ❖ Brown sugar - packed (.5 cup)
- ❖ Egg (1 large)
- ❖ Quick-cooking oats (1.25 cups)
- ❖ Baking soda (.5 tsp.)

Preparation Technique:

1. Warm the oven to reach 350° F/177 ° C. Grease baking trays.
2. Combine the brown sugar and peanut butter, mixing until fluffy.
3. Whisk and mix in the egg. Fold in the oats and baking soda to the creamed mixture.
4. Thoroughly combine and drop by tablespoonfuls two inches apart onto the prepared cookie trays.
5. Flatten each one slightly. Bake for six to eight minutes and cool over wire racks. Store them in a cookie jar.

Peanut Butter Cookies

Servings Provided: 12

Time Required: 1 hour

Macro Counts - Each Serving:

- ❖ Based on 12 cookies:
- ❖ Calories: 140
- ❖ Carbs: 4 g
- ❖ Fiber: 1.2 g
- ❖ Chol: 15.4 mg
- ❖ Protein: 5.8 g
- ❖ Sodium: 134.3 mg
- ❖ Fat Content: 10.4 g (Sat. Fat: 2.1 g)
- ❖ Net Carbs: 2.8 g

Ingredients Needed:

- ❖ Peanut butter - smooth with no-added-sugar (1 cup/250 g)
- ❖ Egg (1 large)
- ❖ Erythritol (.66 or 2/3 cup/135 g)
- ❖ Baking soda (.5 tsp.)
- ❖ Vanilla essence (.5 tsp.)
- ❖ Suggested: Nutribullet or another high-power blender

Preparation Technique:

1. Warm the oven to 350° Fahrenheit/177 ° Celsius.
2. Line a baking tray using a layer of parchment baking paper. Set aside.
3. Pulse the erythritol in a blender until it's powdered. Place it to the side for now. (If you are using a low-carb confectioner's sweetener, you can omit this step).
4. Toss each of the fixings into a mixing container, whisking until a glossy dough is created.
5. Make the balls by rolling about two tablespoons of dough between your palms to form a ball. Put it on the prepared tray. Continue the process until all of the dough has been used (1 dozen cookies)

6. Flatten the cookies using a fork to create a criss-cross pattern across the tops.

7. Bake the cookies for 11-15 minutes.

8. Transfer them to the countertop to cool for ½ hour on the cookie sheet. At that point, transfer the cookies onto a cooling rack for another 15 minutes to ensure they are cooled before storing.

Peanut Butter & Chocolate Kiss Cookies

Servings Provided: 2.5 dozen

Time Required: ½ hour + cooling time

Macro Counts - Each Serving:

- ❖ Calories: 102
- ❖ Carbs: 11 g
- ❖ Sugar: 10 g
- ❖ Fiber: 1 g
- ❖ Prot.: 2 g
- ❖ Sodium: 43 mg
- ❖ Chol: 7 mg
- ❖ Fat Content: 6 g (Saturated: 2 g)

Ingredients Needed:

- ❖ Peanut butter (1 cup)
- ❖ Unchilled egg (1 large)
- ❖ Sugar (1 cup)
- ❖ Vanilla extract (1 tsp.)
- ❖ Milk chocolate kisses (30)

Preparation Technique:

1. Warm the oven to reach 350° Fahrenheit/177 ° Celsius.
2. Cream the sugar with the peanut butter until it's fluffy and light. Whisk the vanilla and egg, mixing it into the batter.
3. Roll the mixture into 1.25-inch balls. Arrange them two inches apart onto ungreased cookie trays. Bake until tops are slightly cracked (10-13 min.).
4. Promptly push one of the chocolate kisses into the center of each cookie.
5. Cool the cookies for about five minutes before removing them from the pans to wire racks.

Simple & Light Cookie Cutouts

Servings Provided: 24

Time Required: 25 minutes

Macro Counts - Each Serving:

- ❖ Calories: 92
- ❖ Carbs: 15 g
- ❖ Fiber: Trace amounts
- ❖ Sodium: 49 mg
- ❖ Protein: 1 g
- ❖ Chol: 14 mg
- ❖ Fat Content: 3 g (Saturated: 1 g)
  D.E.:
- ❖ Starch: 1
- ❖ Fat: ½

Ingredients Needed:

- ❖ Unchilled butter (.25 cup)
- ❖ Sugar (.5 cup)
- ❖ Brown sugar - packed (.5 cup)
- ❖ Canola oil (2 tbsp.)
- ❖ Egg (1)
- ❖ Vanilla extract (.25 tsp.)
- ❖ A.P. flour (1.5 cups)
- ❖ Salt (.25 tsp.)
- ❖ Baking soda (.125 tsp.)
- ❖ Variety Options:
- ❖ Yellow and red food coloring
- ❖ Beaten egg white
- ❖ Popsicle or lollipop sticks

Preparation Technique:

1. Beat the butter with both types of sugars until crumbly (2 min.). Whisk and mix in the egg, oil, and vanilla. Whisk the flour with the salt and baking soda. Slowly add to the mixture.
2. Lightly flour a work surface and divide the dough in half.
3. Roll one piece of the dough into 1/4-inch thickness.
4. Cut with a floured three-inch ghost-shaped (or your favorite) cookie cutter. Arrange the cookies one inch apart on baking sheets coated with cooking spray. Repeat until all of the dough is used.
5. Bake at 350° Fahrenheit or 177 ° Celsius until set (5-6 min.). Cool the cookies for one minute before removing from the pans to wire racks.
6. Decorate as desired.

Vanilla Meringue Cookies

Servings Provided: 5 dozen

Time Required: 1 hour + standing time

Macro Counts - Each Serving:

- ❖ Calories: 10
- ❖ Carbs: 2 g
- ❖ Sugar: 2 g
- ❖ Sodium: 5 mg
- ❖ Fat Content: -0- g
  D.E.:
- ❖ **Free Food**: 1

Ingredients Needed:

- ❖ Egg whites (3 large)
- ❖ Clear/regular vanilla extract (1.5 tsp.)
- ❖ Salt (1 dash)
- ❖ Cream of tartar (.25 tsp.)
- ❖ Sugar (2/3 cup)
- ❖ Useful: Electric mixer

Preparation Technique:

1. Separate and add the egg whites in a small cup and wait for ½ hour until they are at room temperature.
2. Set the oven temperature to 250° F/121° C.
3. Whisk the salt, vanilla, and cream of tartar into the egg whites, beating using the medium-speed setting until foamy.
4. Slowly mix in the sugar (1 tbsp. @ a time), mixing using the high setting after each addition until the sugar is liquified. Continue to beat it to make stiff glossy peaks (7 min.).
5. Use a pastry bag or cut a small hole in the corner of a "food-safe" plastic bag. Insert a #32-star tip. Transfer the meringue into the bag and pipe 1.25-inch-diameter cookies - two inches apart onto parchment-lined baking sheets.

6. Bake until firm to the touch (40-45 min.).

7. Turn the power off to the oven. Leave the meringues in the warm oven for one hour (oven door closed). Transfer them from the oven and thoroughly cool on the baking trays.

8. Transfer the meringues from the paper and store them in an airtight container at room temperature.

Chapter 11

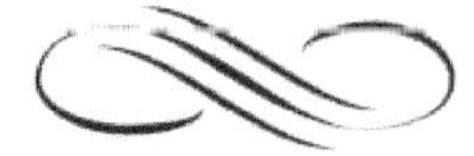

Snack Bars

Almond Espresso Bars

Servings Provided: 4 dozen

Time Required: 35 minutes + cool time

Macro Counts - Each Serving:

- ❖ Calories: 68
- ❖ Carbs: 11 g
- ❖ Fiber: -0- g
- ❖ Sugar: 8 g
- ❖ Chol: 7 mg
- ❖ Prot.: 1 g
- ❖ Sodium: 55 mg
- ❖ Fat Content: 2 g (Saturated: 1 g)
  D.E.:
- ❖ Starch: 1
- ❖ Fat: ½

Ingredients Needed:

- ❖ Unchilled butter (.25 cup)
- ❖ Brown sugar - packed (1 cup)
- ❖ Brewed espresso (.5 cup)
- ❖ Egg (1 large)

- ❖ Self-rising flour (1.5 cups)
- ❖ Chopped slivered almonds - toasted (.75 cup)
- ❖ Ground cinnamon (.5 tsp.)
- ❖ The Glaze:
- ❖ Confectioners' sugar (1.5 cups)
- ❖ Water (3 tbsp.)
- ❖ Almond extract (.75 tsp.)
- ❖ Slivered almonds - toasted (.25 cup)
- ❖ Needed: 15x10x1-in. baking pan

Preparation Technique:

1. Mix the butter with the brown sugar and espresso until blended. Whisk and mix in the egg. Whisk the flour with the cinnamon, slowly adding it to the creamed mixture. Chop and stir in the almonds.
2. Spread them onto a greased baking pan. Bake at 350° Fahrenheit or 177 ° Celsius until lightly browned (18-22 min.).
3. In another mixing container, combine the water with the confectioners' sugar and extract until creamy smooth.
4. Spread the mixture over warm bars with a sprinkle with slivered almonds. Cool on a wire rack.
5. Slice them into bars to serve.

Cherry-Almond Cheesecake Bars

Servings Provided: 20

Time Required: 3 hours

Macro Counts - Each Serving:

- Calories: 141
- Carbs: 13.5 g
- Sugar: 7.8 g
- Fiber: 0.6 g
- Chol: 22.9 mg
- Prot.: 4.3 g
- Sodium: 116.2 mg
- Fat Content: 8 g (Saturated: 4.4 g)
  D.E.:
- Fat: 1 ½
- Other Carbohydrate: 1

Ingredients Needed:

- Packed brown sugar (3 tbsp.)
- Almonds - finely chopped (2 tbsp.)
- A.P. flour (.66 cup)
- Rolled oats - quick-cooking (.66 cup)
- Butter (.25 cup)
- Reduced-fat cream cheese - Neufchatel (2 - 8 oz. pkg.)
- Granulated sugar (1/3 cup)
- Vanilla (2 tsp.)
- Almond extract (.25 tsp.)
- Refrigerated/frozen egg product, thawed,(1 cup) or Eggs (4)
- Dried cherries (1/3 cup)
- Optional: F.F. frozen whipped dessert topping (10 tbsp.)
- Optional: Sliced almonds (2 tbsp.)
- Suggested: 8x8x2-inch baking pan

Preparation Technique:

1. Set the oven temperature at 350° F/177 ° C.
2. Thaw the topping.
3. Lightly grease the baking tray or cover it using a foil layer, extending it up and over the edges of the pan. Place it to the side for now.
4. Combine the flour with brown sugar, almonds, and oats.
5. Work or cut in the butter using a pastry blender until it is a bunch of coarse crumbs. Use your hands and push the crumbs into the bottom of the pan.
6. Set a timer to bake for 12 minutes.
7. Beat the cream cheese with the vanilla extract, granulated sugar, and almond extract using an electric mixer on the medium speed setting until it's 'fluffy' and light. Slowly mix in the egg, combining it on the low-speed setting - just until incorporated.
8. Finely chop and stir in the cherries. Spread the cream cheese mixture over the partially baked crust.
9. Bake until the cream cheese layer is set (25-35 min.). Thoroughly cool in the pan on a wire rack. Place a layer of plastic wrap over them and chill for two to 24 hours before serving.
10. Slice them into bars to serve, adding dessert topping or almonds to your liking.
11. Store them in the fridge to keep them fresh.

Chocolate-Pumpkin Cheesecake Bars

Servings Provided: 24

Time Required: 50 minutes

Macro Counts - Each Serving:

- ❖ Calories: 197
- ❖ Carbs: 29 g
- ❖ Sugar: 19 g
- ❖ Fiber: 2 g
- ❖ Chol: 40 mg
- ❖ Prot.: 4 g
- ❖ Sodium: 157 mg
- ❖ Fat Content: 8 g (Saturated: 5 g)
  D.E.:
- ❖ Starch: 2
- ❖ Fat: 1

Ingredients Needed:

- ❖ Butter - cubed (1/3 cup)
- ❖ Unsweetened chocolate (1.5 oz.)
- ❖ Boiling water (.5 cup)
- ❖ Instant coffee granules (1 tbsp.)
- ❖ Canned pumpkin (1 cup)
- ❖ Eggs - whisked (2 large)
- ❖ Sugar (1.5 cups)
- ❖ A.P. flour (2 cups)
- ❖ Baking soda (.75 tsp.)
- ❖ Salt (.5 tsp.)
- ❖ The Batter:
- ❖ Reduced-fat cream cheese (8 oz. pkg.)
- ❖ Canned pumpkin (.5 cup)
- ❖ Vanilla extract (1 tsp.)

- ❖ Sugar (.25 cup)
- ❖ Ground cloves (.125 tsp.)
- ❖ Cinnamon (.75 tsp.)
- ❖ Ground ginger (.75 tsp.)
- ❖ Egg - lightly beaten (1 large)
- ❖ Semisweet chocolate chips (1 cup)
- ❖ Needed: 15x10x1-inch baking pan

Preparation Technique:

1. Coarsely chop the chocolate.
2. Melt the butter with the chocolate in the microwave, stirring until smooth. Cool slightly.
3. Use a big mixing container, liquify the coffee in water, and mix in the eggs, pumpkin, and chocolate mixture.
4. Whisk the flour with the sugar, baking soda, and salt. Slowly add it to the chocolate mixture. Transfer to the baking pan coated with cooking oil spray.
5. Prepare the cheesecake batter in a mixing container.
6. Combine and mix the pumpkin with the cream cheese until smooth.
7. Fold in the vanilla, sugar, and spices. Whisk and add the egg, beating using the low-speed setting until barely incorporated.
8. Spoon the mixture over the chocolate batter. Swirl the mixture using a knife to mix the cheesecake portion. Sprinkle with chocolate chips.
9. Bake at 350° Fahrenheit or 177 ° Celsius until a toothpick inserted in the center comes out with moist crumbs (20-25 min.). Cool on a wire rack.
10. Cut into bars and refrigerate any leftovers.

Chocolate-Drizzled Peanut Butter Cheesecake Bars

Servings Provided: 24

Time Required: ½ hour

Macro Counts - Each Serving:

- ❖ Calories: 145
- ❖ Carbs: 13 g
- ❖ Fiber: 1 g
- ❖ Sugar: 8 g
- ❖ Chol: 8 mg
- ❖ Prot.: 7 g
- ❖ Sodium: 203 mg
- ❖ Fat Content: g (Saturated: g)
  D.E.:
- ❖ Starch: 1
- ❖ Fat: 1
- ❖ Fruit: 1
- ❖ Lean Meat: 1

Ingredients Needed:

- ❖ Nonstick cooking spray (as needed)
- ❖ Rolled oats - regular cut (.5 cup)
- ❖ Whole wheat flour (.5 cup)
- ❖ Brown sugar - tightly packed (.25 cup)
- ❖ Butter - melted (.25 cup)
- ❖ Unchilled - F.F. cream cheese (2 - 8 oz. pkg.)
- ❖ Creamy peanut butter (.75 cup)
- ❖ Granulated sugar (.33 cup)
- ❖ Refrigerated/frozen egg product - thawed (.75 cup)
- ❖ F.F. milk (.25 cup + 2 tbsp.)
- ❖ Vanilla (1 tsp.)
- ❖ Semisweet chocolate - chopped (2 oz.)

- ❖ Chopped peanuts (3 tbsp.)
- ❖ Cooking oil spray (as needed)
- ❖ Needed: 13x9x2-inch baking pan

Preparation Technique:

1. Warm the oven to reach 350° F/177 ° C.
2. Spritz the pan using a portion of the oil spray.
3. Measure and toss the oats into a blender/food processor. Securely close the lid and pulse until they are coarsely ground.
4. Toss the ground oats with the brown sugar, flour, and melted butter. Evenly press it into the base of the baking tray.
5. Mix the granulated sugar with the cream cheese and peanut butter, using an electric mixer until combined (medium-speed setting). Pour in ¼ cup of milk, vanilla, and egg substitute. Mix it using the low-speed setting - just until combined.
6. Empty the filling into the prepared crust. Set a timer and bake until set in the center (25 min.).
7. Cool the bars in the pan for ½ hour. Put a layer of foil over the top of the pan. Pop it into the fridge for a minimum of four hours or up to 24 hours.
8. Use a heavy saucepan to melt the chocolate using the low-temperature setting until melted. Transfer the pan to a cool spot and mix in enough milk (2-3 tbsp.) to make it a drizzling consistency.
9. Empty the melted chocolate into a small resealable plastic bag. Seal the bag and snip off a small corner from the bag. Pipe the chocolate over the cheesecake. Sprinkle with chopped peanuts and cover with plastic wrap to cool. Serve when it's set.

Layered Pumpkin Cheesecake Bars

Servings Provided: 16

Time Required: 50 minutes + chill time

Macro Counts - Each Serving:

- ❖ Calories: 117
- ❖ Carbs: 13 g
- ❖ Fiber: -0- g
- ❖ Sugar: 9 g
- ❖ Chol: 31 mg
- ❖ Prot.: 3 g
- ❖ Sodium: 135 mg
- ❖ Fat Content: 6 g (Saturated:4 g)
  D.E.:
- ❖ Fat: 1
- ❖ Starch: 1

Ingredients Needed:

- ❖ Graham cracker crumbs (1 cup)
- ❖ Melted butter - reduced-fat (2 tbsp.)
- ❖ Sugar (2 tbsp.)
- ❖ The Filling:
- ❖ R.F. cream cheese (11 oz.)
- ❖ R.F. sour cream (.33 cup)
- ❖ Sugar (.33 cup)
- ❖ A.P. flour (2 tsp.)
- ❖ Vanilla extract (.5 tsp.)
- ❖ Egg (1 large)
- ❖ Brown sugar (1 tbsp.)
- ❖ Pumpkin from a can (.5 cup)
- ❖ Also Suggested: 9-inch baking dish

Preparation Technique:

1. Toss the sugar with the cracker crumbs. Add in the butter. Press onto the bottom of the dish coated with a spritz of cooking oil spray.
2. Bake at 325° Fahrenheit or 163° Celsius until set (6-10 min.). Remove and place them onto a rack to cool.
3. Prepare the filling in a big mixing container. Mix the sour cream with the cream cheese, flour, sugar, and vanilla until it's creamy smooth. Whisk and mix in the egg, beating on the low setting - just until combined.
4. Remove 3/4 cup of the batter to a mixing container, and fold in brown sugar and pumpkin until thoroughly mixed.
5. Pour plain batter over the crust. Next, spread pumpkin batter over plain batter.
6. Bake at 325° Fahrenheit or 163° Celsius until the center is almost set (20-25 min.).
7. Next, wait for it to cool for one hour on a wire rack.
8. Place a layer of foil or plastic wrap over the bars and pop the pan into the fridge for at least two hours.

Light & Easy Cheesecake Bars

Servings Provided: 1.5 dozen

Time Required: 50 minutes + chill time

Macro Counts - Each Serving:

- ❖ Calories: 153
- ❖ Carbs: 19 g
- ❖ Fiber: -0- g
- ❖ Sugar: 12 g
- ❖ Chol: 31 mg
- ❖ Prot.: 4 g
- ❖ Sodium: 216 mg
- ❖ Fat Content: 7 g (Saturated: 4 g)
  D.E.:
- ❖ Starch: 1
- ❖ Fat: 1 ½

Ingredients Needed:

- ❖ Unchilled butter - softened (1/3 cup)
- ❖ Lemon juice - divided (4 tbsp.)
- ❖ A.P. flour (1.25 cups)
- ❖ Sugar - divided (1 cup)
- ❖ Salt (.5 tsp.)
- ❖ Cream cheese - reduced-fat (8 oz. pkg.)
- ❖ Cream cheese - fat-free (8 oz. pkg.)
- ❖ Egg (1 large)
- ❖ Grated lemon zest (2 tsp.)
- ❖ Raspberries (18 fresh - halved)
- ❖ Needed: 9-inch square pan

Preparation Technique:

1. Line the baking pan with foil and coat with a spritz of cooking oil spray. Place the pan to the side for now.
2. Mix the butter with ¼ cup sugar until smooth (2 min.). Stir in two tablespoons lemon juice. Mix in the flour and salt. Press into the covered pan.
3. Bake at 350° Fahrenheit or 177 ° Celsius until the edges are nicely browned (14-16 min.).
4. Meanwhile, combine the cream cheeses and remaining sugar until smooth. Add in the whisked egg, beating using the low-speed setting just until combined. Mix in lemon zest and the rest of the lemon juice. Empty it over the crust.
5. Bake until filling is set (14-18 min.).
6. Let it cool on a wire rack for one hour. Pop it into the fridge for about two hours. Using foil, lift bars out of the pan. Gently peel off the layer of foil and cut them into squares, then triangles. Top it off using the raspberries.

Chapter 12

Candy & Other Tasty Favorites

Servings Provided: 15

Time Required: 10 minutes

Macro Counts - Each Serving:

- ❖ Calories: 70
- ❖ Carbs: 9 g
- ❖ Sugar: 6 g
- ❖ Fiber: 1 g
- ❖ Chol: 1 mg
- ❖ Prot.: 3 g
- ❖ Sodium: 46 mg
- ❖ Fat Content: 3 g (Saturated: 1 g)
  D.E.:
- ❖ Starch: ½
- ❖ Fat: ½

Ingredients Needed:

- ❖ Chunky peanut butter (.33 cup)
- ❖ Honey (.25 cup)
- ❖ Vanilla extract (.5 tsp.)
- ❖ Quick-cooking oats (.33 cup)

* Nonfat dry milk powder (.33 cup)
* Graham cracker crumbs (2 tbsp.)

Preparation Technique:

1. Cream the peanut butter with the honey and vanilla. Mix in the milk powder, oats, and cracker crumbs.
2. Shape the mixture into one-inch balls. Cover and pop them into the fridge until it's time to serve.

Peppermint Meringues

Servings Provided: 1.5 dozen

Time Required: 1 hour 40 minutes + cool time

Macro Counts - Each Serving:

- ❖ Calories: 32
- ❖ Carbs: 8 g
- ❖ Sugar: 7 g
- ❖ Chol: -0- mg
- ❖ Sodium: 23 mg
- ❖ Fat Content: -0- g
  D.E.:
- ❖ Starch: ½

Ingredients Needed:

- ❖ Egg whites, room temperature (2 large)
- ❖ Salt (.125 tsp.)
- ❖ Sugar (.5 cup)
- ❖ Cream of tartar (.125 tsp.)
- ❖ Peppermint candy canes (2 crushed)

Preparation Technique:

1. Beat the egg whites until foamy. Sprinkle in the cream of tartar and salt, mixing until you reach the soft peak stage.
2. Slowly mix in the sugar to reach stiff peaks (7 min.). Drop the mixture by teaspoonfuls onto paper or foil-lined baking sheets. Decorate them using the crushed candy.
3. Bake at 225° Fahrenheit or 107° Celsius for 1.5 hours.
4. Extinguish the oven's heat and leave the cookies with the door slightly open until cooled (1 hr.).
5. Keep them in a closed container.

Sour Cream Bavarian

Servings Provided: 8 (1.25 cups sauce)

Time Required: 15 minutes + chill time

Macro Counts - Each Serving:

- ❖ Calories: 176
- ❖ Carbs: 33 g
- ❖ Fiber: 2 g
- ❖ Sugar: 30 g
- ❖ Chol: 1 mg
- ❖ Fat Content: -0- g (Saturated: -0- g)
- ❖ Sodium: 37 mg
- ❖ Protein: 3 g

Ingredients Needed:

- ❖ Unflavored gelatin (1 envelope)
- ❖ Water - cold (.75 cup)
- ❖ Sugar (.66 cup)
- ❖ Vanilla extract (1 tsp.)
- ❖ Sour cream - fat-free (1 cup)
- ❖ Whipped topping - fat-free (2 cups)
- ❖ The Sauce:
- ❖ Frozen sweetened raspberries or sliced strawberries - thawed (10 oz. pkg.)
- ❖ Cornstarch (1 tbsp.)
- ❖ Sugar (1 tbsp.)

Preparation Technique:

1. Prepare a saucepan, and sprinkle the gelatin into cold water. Wait for one minute. Add sugar and warm it while stirring using the low-temperature setting until the gelatin and sugar are liquified.

2. Transfer the mixture into a bowl. Whisk in sour cream and vanilla and refrigerate it for ten minutes.

3. Mix in the whipped topping. Empty it into a four-cup mold coated with cooking spray. Refrigerate, covered, until firm, about four hours.
4. Prepare the sauce by draining the berries, reserving the syrup. Pour in enough water to the syrup to measure ¾ cup.
5. Use a small saucepan to mix the cornstarch with the sugar and syrup mixture until smooth. Once boiling, simmer and stir until thickened (2 min.). Cool slightly. Stir in drained berries and refrigerate until serving.
6. To serve, unmold dessert onto a serving plate. Serve with sauce.

Keto-Friendly Fat Bombs

Chocolate Bombs

Servings Provided: 12

Time Required: 25 minutes

Macro Counts - Each Serving:

- ❖ Calories: 194
- ❖ Carbs: 3.5 g
- ❖ Fiber: 1.5 g
- ❖ Sugar: 0.3 g
- ❖ Chol: 3.2 mg
- ❖ Protein: 3.8 g
- ❖ Sodium: 1.1 mg
- ❖ Fat Content: 16.8 g (Saturated: 10 g)
- ❖ Net Carbs: 2 g

Ingredients Needed:

- ❖ Unsweetened Cacao/cocoa powder (.25 cup/21 g)
- ❖ Natural chunky peanut butter (5 tbsp.)
- ❖ Shelled hemp seeds (6 tbsp.)
- ❖ Heavy cream (2 tbsp.)
- ❖ Unchilled-unrefined coconut oil (.5 cup/100 g)
- ❖ Vanilla extract (1 tsp.)
- ❖ Stevia (2 tbsp.)

Preparation Technique:

1. Mix the cocoa powder with the hemp seeds and peanut butter in a large mixing container.
2. Mix in the oil until it is pasty. Fold in the vanilla, stevia, and cream - sitting until it's a paste once again.
3. Roll the mixture into balls. (If the paste is too thin to roll, pop it in the fridge for ½ hour before proceeding.) Roll them in shredded coconut.
4. Arrange the balls on a layer of parchment baking paper on a cookie tin.

5. Freeze for ten minutes or leave them in the fridge for a minimum of 30 minutes before serving.

Peanut Butter Bombs

Servings Provided: 12

Time Required: 10 minutes prep - 1 .5 hours wait time

Macro Counts - Per Serving:

- ½ bomb = 1 serving:
- Calories: 247
- Carbohydrates: 247 g
- Sugar: 0.5 g
- Fiber: 1.2 g
- Prot.: 3.6 g
- Chol: -0- mg
- Sodium: 101.7 mg
- Fat Content: 24.4 g (Saturated: 15.3 g)

Ingredients Needed:

- The Bombs:
- Coconut oil (.5 cup/100 g)
- Peanut butter - no added salt or sugar (.75 cup/185 g)
- Sea salt (.25 tsp.)
- Vanilla extract (1 tsp.)
- Liquid stevia (3-4 drops)
- The Ganache:
- Cocoa powder (1 tbsp.)
- Coconut oil (6 tbsp.)
- Liquid stevia/favorite sweetener (1-2 drops)
- Also Needed: Six-count muffin tray

Preparation Technique:

1. Use a small bowl to melt the coconut oil and combine it with the peanut butter, stevia sweetener, vanilla extract, and salt. Heat in the microwave briefly and whisk until creamy.

2. Prepare the muffin tray with paper cups. Spoon the peanut butter mixture into each cup (3 tbsp. each).
3. Pop them in the fridge for at least one hour to overnight until firm.
4. Meanwhile, whisk the ganache ingredients until smooth.
5. Spoon about one tablespoon of the ganache over each fat bomb.
6. Chill for at least 30 minutes in the fridge before serving.
7. Enjoy them for up to one week stored in the fridge.

Chapter 13

Beverages

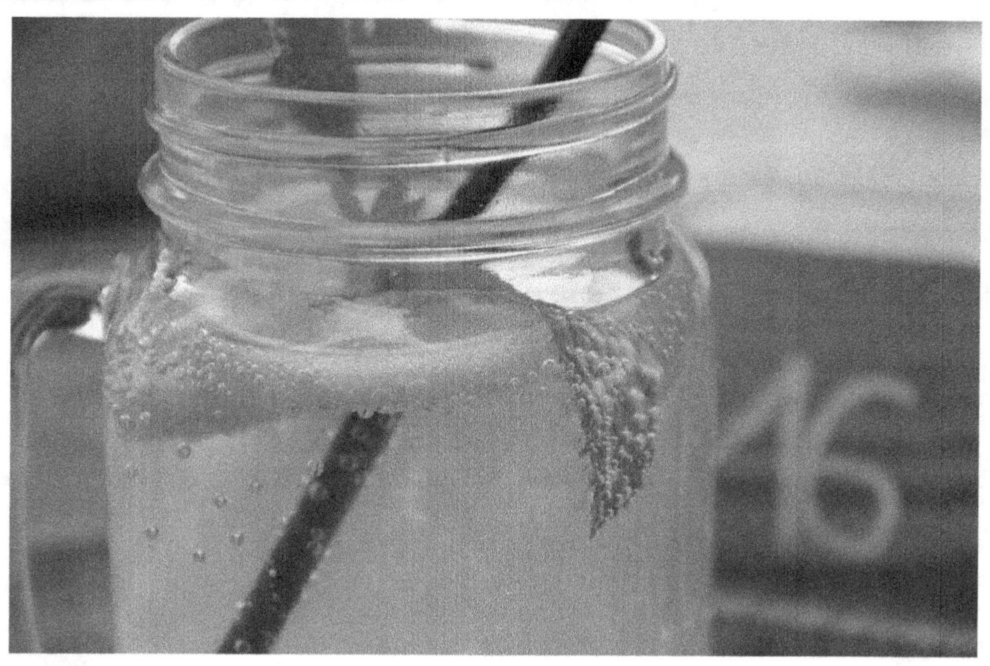

Basil Lemonade

Servings Provided: 6

Time Required: 20 minutes

Macro Counts - Each Serving:

- ❖ ¾ cup portion:
- ❖ Calories: 98
- ❖ Fiber: 0.3 g
- ❖ Carbs: 26.8 g
- ❖ Sugar: 24.3 g
- ❖ Prot.: 0.5 g

- ❖ Sodium: 5.5 mg
- ❖ Fat Content: 0.2 g
  D.E.:
- ❖ Other Carbohydrate: 1 ½

Ingredients Needed:

- ❖ Fresh lemon juice (1.25 cups/+ more for garnishing/from about 8 lemons)
- ❖ Honey/agave syrup (.5 cup)
- ❖ Packed fresh basil leaves (1 cup + more to garnish)
- ❖ Water (3 cups - cold)
- ❖ Ice cubes (1 cup)

Preparation Technique:

- ❖ Load the blender with the basil, honey, and lemon juice, mixing until it's creamy smooth. Pour it into a large jar or pitcher using a sieve to strain.
- ❖ Pour in the water and pop it into the fridge until time to serve.
- ❖ Enjoy it over ice and a lemon slice with a couple of basil leaves.

Citrus Spa Water

Servings Provided: 6

Time Required: 5 minutes

Macro Counts - Each Serving:

- ❖ Calories: 23
- ❖ Sugar: 2 g
- ❖ Sodium: 10 mg
- ❖ Net Carbs: 6 g

Ingredients Needed:

- ❖ Lemon (1)
- ❖ Lime (1)
- ❖ Orange (1)
- ❖ Pink grapefruit (1)
- ❖ Water (6 cups)

Preparation Technique:

1. Slice each piece of fruit into halves.
2. Juice all of the fruit into a measuring cup and trash the rinds.
3. Pour the juice through a strainer and into a pitcher that will hold at least 8 cups of liquid.
4. Add the water and stir well to serve.

Fruit Sparklers

Servings Provided: 6

Time Required: 5 minutes

Macro Counts - Each Serving:

- ❖ Calories: 23
- ❖ Carbs: 6 g
- ❖ Sugar: 5.5 g
- ❖ Sodium: 38.7 mg
  D.E.: Fruit: ½

Ingredients Needed:

- ❖ Ice cubes (1 cup)
- ❖ Low-calorie grape/cranberry or pomegranate juice (3 cups)
- ❖ Sparkling water (3 cups)
- ❖ Optional: Halved fresh cranberries, grapes, or raspberries (.75 cup)

Preparation Technique:

1. Half fill six tall glasses with ice cubes.
2. Portion the grape juice evenly between the glasses.
3. Pour sparkling water into the glasses, and gently stir.
4. Decorate with a few floating grapes in the drinks.

Ginger-Lemon Tea

Servings Provided: 5

Time Required: 20 minutes

Macro Counts - Each Serving:

- ❖ Calories: 3
- ❖ Protein: 0.5 g
- ❖ Sodium: 2.9mg
- ❖ Saturated: -0- g
- ❖ Free exchanges

Ingredients Needed:

- ❖ Water (6 cups)
- ❖ Sugar substitute (1 tbsp.)
- ❖ Lemon peel (8 strips)
- ❖ Fresh ginger (2-inch piece)
- ❖ Green tea bags (3)
- ❖ Lemon (5 slices)

Preparation Technique:

1. Slice the lemon strips (2.5 x 1-inches). Peel and thinly slice the ginger.
2. Prepare a saucepan of water and toss in the strips of lemon and ginger. Lower the temperature setting, and simmer for ten minutes. Discard the ginger and lemon.
3. Toss the tea bags in a teapot and promptly add to the simmering lemon-infused water. Place a lid on the pot and steep for one to three minutes. Remove the tea bags, squeezing gently.
4. Serve right away in heatproof glass mugs or cups. Sweeten as desired using your favorite sugar substitute and serve with lemon slices.
5. Tip: Remove lemon peel with a vegetable peeler. If necessary, use a sharp knife to scrape off any white pith that remains on the peel, as this can cause bitterness.

Peach Sunrise Refresher

Servings Provided: 4

Time Required: 5 minutes

Macro Counts - Each Serving:

- ❖ Calories: 47
- ❖ Fiber: 0.5 g
- ❖ Sugar: 11.7 g
- ❖ Carbs: 0.2 g
- ❖ Chol: -0- mg
- ❖ Sodium: 24.3 mg
- ❖ Fat Content: -0- g
- ❖ D.E.: Other Carbohydrate: 1

Ingredients Needed:

- ❖ Ice - divided (2 cups)
- ❖ Diet cranberry juice drink - divided (1.33 cups)
- ❖ Peach nectar, divided (1.33 cups)
- ❖ Mint (4 sprigs)
- ❖ Quartered orange (4 slices)

Preparation Technique:

1. Put ½ cup of ice into each of the glasses.
2. Add 1/3 cup portions of cranberry juice and peach nectar to each glass.
3. Top them off with mint springs and orange slices.

Strawberry Água Fresca

Servings Provided: 6 cups

Time Required: 5 minutes

Macro Counts - Each Serving:

- ❖ Calories: 16
- ❖ Fiber: 1 g
- ❖ Carbs: 4 g
- ❖ Sugar: 3 g
- ❖ Sodium: 30 mg
- ❖ Fat Content: -0- g
- ❖ Prot.: 0.3 g
- ❖ Net Carbs: 3 g

Ingredients Needed:

- ❖ Fresh strawberries (2 cups)
- ❖ Water (4 cups)
- ❖ Kosher salt (1 pinch)
- ❖ Optional: Honey or another sweetener (1 tbsp.)

Preparation Technique:

1. Place the strawberries, water, salt, and sweetener into a blender.
2. Purée until smooth.
3. Serve in chilled glasses.

Diabetic-Friendly Cocktails & Mocktails

Blood Orange Margaritas

Servings Provided: 6

Time Required: 15 minutes

Macro Counts - Each Serving:

- Calories: 152
- Fiber: 0.3 g
- Carbs: 12.6g
- Sugar: 9.8 g
- Prot.: 0.4 g
- Sodium: 1.9 mg
- Fat Content: 0.1 g (Saturated: -0- g)
  D.E.:
- Alcohol Equivalent: 1
- Fruit: ½

Ingredients Needed:

- Grated blood orange zest (1 tbsp.)
- Optional: Kosher salt (1 tbsp.)
- Blood orange juice (1 cup)
- White tequila (1 cup)
- Lime juice (.5 cup + 1 lime wedge)
- Triple Sec (.25 cup)
- Simple syrup (2 tbsp.)
- Ice cubes (1 cup)
- To Garnish:
- Blood orange slices (6 slices)
- Lime slices (12 slices)

Preparation Technique:

1. Chill the tequila and orange juice.

2. Sprinkle orange zest on a small plate and combine with salt (if using).

3. Mix the tequila with the lime juice, simple syrup, orange juice, and Triple Sec in a pitcher.

4. Rub the rims of six glasses with the lime wedge and dip in the zest (or zest-salt mixture).

5. Fill each of the glasses with ice and pour in about ½ cup of the margarita mixture into each. Top it off with lime or orange slices as desired.

Hot Cider with Apple Brandy & Spices

Servings Provided: 8

Time Required: 25 minutes

Macro Counts - Each Serving:

- ❖ Calories: 184
- ❖ Carbs: 30 g
- ❖ Sugar: 29 g
- ❖ Sodium: 0.3 mg
- ❖ Fat Content: -0- g
- ❖ **D.E.:**
- ❖ Fruit: 2

Ingredients Needed:

- ❖ Apple cider/apple juice (8 cups)
- ❖ Whole allspice berries (4)
- ❖ Whole cloves (4)
- ❖ Whole cardamom seeds (4)
- ❖ Cinnamon (4 sticks)
- ❖ Calvados - brandy (1 cup)

Preparation Technique:

1. Combine the cider or juice with the cloves, cardamom, allspice, and cinnamon sticks in a large saucepan.
2. Simmer for 20 minutes and strain out the spices
3. Stir in the Calvados or brandy.
4. Serve piping-hot in heavy mugs.

Hot Cocoa & Bourbon

Servings Provided: 6

Time Required: 15 minutes

Macro Counts - Each Serving:

- ❖ 2/3 Cup Cocoa & 1.5 Tablespoons Topper:
- ❖ Calories: 203
- ❖ Carbs: 23.5 g
- ❖ Fiber: 2.1 g
- ❖ Sugar: 19.8 g
- ❖ Chol: 3.3 mg
- ❖ Prot.: 7.2 g
- ❖ Sodium: 69.8 mg
- ❖ Fat Content: 6.3 g (Saturated: 3.7 g)
  D.E.:
- ❖ Starch: ½
- ❖ Fat: 2
- ❖ Other Carbohydrate: ½
- ❖ Milk: ½

Ingredients Needed:

- ❖ Bittersweet chocolate pieces (.5 cup)
- ❖ Unsweetened cocoa powder (.25 cup)
- ❖ Fat-free milk (4 cups)
- ❖ Honey (2 tbsp.)
- ❖ Bourbon (.5 cup/4 oz.)
- ❖ Ground cinnamon (1 pinch)

Preparation Technique:

1. Melt the chocolate pieces and cocoa powder in a saucepan.
2. Whisk in 3.5 cups of the milk and the honey.

3. Simmer using the medium-temperature setting, just until boiling and chocolate pieces are melted, whisking constantly. Stir in the bourbon.
4. For a frothy topper, pour the rest of the milk (.5 cup) into a medium bowl. Microwave 20-30 seconds or until warm. Beat with a whisk until frothy.
5. Serve the cocoa with a frothy topper and a sprinkle of cinnamon or more cocoa powder.

Mojito Mocktails

Servings Provided: 4

Time Required: 10 minutes

Macro Counts - Each Serving:

- ❖ Calories: 124
- ❖ Carbs: 33.5 g
- ❖ Sugar: 26.5 g
- ❖ Prot.: 0.8 g
- ❖ Fat Content: 0.2 g (Saturated: -0- g)
- ❖ Sodium: 6.1 mg
- ❖ D.E.:Starch: Other Carbohydrate: 1 ½

Ingredients Needed:

- ❖ Fresh lime juice (.75 cup/from 6 limes)
- ❖ Simple syrup (.75 cup **)
- ❖ Packed fresh mint leaves (.5 cup)
- ❖ Lime zest (2 strips - 2-inch)
- ❖ Ice cubes (4 cups)
- ❖ Sparkling water (2 cups)
- ❖ To Garnish: Lime slices (4 slices @ ¼-inch thickness) & mint sprigs (4)

Preparation Technique:

1. Make your simple syrup: **Pour one cup of sugar into a medium saucepan, frequently stirring until it's liquified. Cool the mixture for ½ hour and refrigerate until cold (1 hr.). Simple syrup can be stored in the fridge, covered, for up to six months.
2. Combine the lime juice, simple syrup, mint leaves, and lime zest in a pitcher. Lightly crush the mint and zest.
3. Add ice cubes and sparkling water, thoroughly stirring to serve.
4. Portion the drink into four glasses. Garnish with lime slices and mint sprigs, as desired.

Snow Banks Sparkling Wine Cocktail

Servings Provided: 1 serving or 1.5 cups

Time Required: 1 hour 40 minutes

Macro Counts - Each Serving:

- ❖ 5 fl oz. portion:
- ❖ Calories: 126
- ❖ Carbs: 11.1 g
- ❖ Sugar: 8.8 g
- ❖ Fiber: 0.1 g
- ❖ Chol: -0- mg
- ❖ Prot.: 0.4 g
- ❖ Sodium: 0.5 mg
- ❖ Fat Content: -0- g
  D.E.:
- ❖ Other Carbohydrates: ½
- ❖ Fat: 2

Ingredients Needed:

- ❖ The Simple Syrup:
- ❖ Sugar (1 cup)
- ❖ Water (1 cup)
- ❖ The Cocktail:
- ❖ Fresh lemon juice (.5 oz.)
- ❖ Chilled sparkling wine - ex. - Prosecco (4 oz.)
- ❖ Simple Syrup ↑ (.5 oz.)
- ❖ To Garnish: 1 Lemon twist

Preparation Technique:

- ❖ Make the simple syrup by bringing the water and sugar to a boil in a saucepan, frequently stirring to liquefy the sugar. Cool it for ½ hour and refrigerate until cold (1 hr.).

❖ To prepare an individual cocktail: Combine ½ oz. of the simple syrup and lemon juice in a champagne flute.

❖ Top it off using sparkling wine and garnish with a lemon twist.

Conclusion

I hope you have thoroughly enjoyed each of the recipes provided in your new copy of the Diabetic Desserts for Beginners I hope it was informative and provided you with all of the tools you need to achieve your goals, whatever they may be.

The next step is to head to the market and prepare one of the delicious options for dessert tonight!

The experts state you don't need to eliminate all sugar. However, many will eventually consume more sugar than is healthy. You need to learn moderation, especially if you have diabetes. Thus, you'll find this cookbook will be your best friend, so you can enjoy your favorite dessert once in a while.

It takes time for your taste buds to adjust once you begin to reduce your intake of sugar. Thus, your cravings should also diminish.

When you want to enjoy dessert, eliminate that portion of pasta, rice, or bread. It is all in working the carbohydrates to your advantage, instead of making it difficult to pack the meal with both options.

Consider adding more healthy fat as you enjoy dessert. Fat will slow down the digestive process, which means your blood sugar levels won't spike quickly. However, you shouldn't reach for the donuts. Envision healthier fats, such as ricotta cheese, yogurt, peanut butter, or nuts.

Save your sweets for mealtime, not a mid-afternoon snack. When eaten solo, sweets will cause your blood sugar to spike. However, if you eat them with other healthy foods as part of your meal, your blood sugar will not rise as rapidly.

Enjoy every morsel of your special dessert dish. Eat slowly and indulge in its flavor. Not only will the food be more enjoyable, but you are also less likely to overeat.

I sincerely hope you have found the information useful. Finally, if you found this book helpful in any way, a review on Amazon is always appreciated!